EMPATH SELF CARE

3 BOOKS IN 1

MASTER THE HIDDEN SECRETS TO HEAL YOURSELF FROM RACIAL TRAUMA, COMPULSIVE BEHAVIORS AND TOXIC RELATIONSHIPS.

PRACTICE MINDFULNESS AND START CARING FOR YOURSELF

ADELE ADANI

"If you want something you never had, you have to do something you've never done"

NARCISSISTIC ABUSE AND CODEPENDENCY

Disarm the malignant narcissist with the ultimate guide to build an unbeatable mind. Break down the hidden gaslighting and escape from a toxic relationship.

ADELE ADANI

PART 1: UNDERSTANDING THE NARCISSIST

What is Narcissistic Personality Disorder (NPD)?

In a nutshell, it can be interpreted as only the interests of the narcissist matter. In comparison, your interests don't matter because they will do whatever it takes to fulfill their needs at your expense due to restricting their capacities and external restrictions. From the victim's viewpoint, it's interpreted as violence. From the narcissist's perspective, it's perceived as simply a normal function, like stretching out a hand to pluck the fruit from the flower; you're the tree. The narcissist's motivation source is the pathology of their uncompromising desires.

What makes the tyrannical demands of the narcissist the next step is disdain. The narcissist is nonsensical unless you consider disdain. We all have desires, so we don't despise others' needs. Narcissists are contemptuous of your desires, they are contemptuous of your weakness, they are contemptuous of the fact that you still have needs, they blame you for getting them, and they strive to harm you with your needs, purposely allowing them to fail. Contempt lifts the narcissist. This ultimately causes them to undermine the trust, as trust is weakness, and vulnerability causes their disdain.

The narcissist has virtually no internal limits on abusing or abusing you unlimitedly, and they have no regard for anything; nothing is holy to the narcissist. The narcissist doesn't take anyone or something seriously because they just disrespect everything, often leading them to feel contempt or indifference about anything they inevitably encounter. They're not shameful for what they're doing, nor should you make them responsible or take responsibilities when they've never taken you seriously. They don't feel shameful or accountable to anyone; they're disdainful or indifferent. They hate your accident and your ability to know the facts. They hate your desires and feelings, disregarding both. Their invalidations often arise from their disdain for being noticed or heard.

Narcissistic assault victims also experience subtle hostility in relationships. This, too, is the product of their hidden idea when they claim to love you. Narcissists may send off a shell of lucidity and reason, but they don't think straight because they still hate reasoning or reality. If you do your homework, you can start finding inconsistencies in their reasoning and contradictions in their statements and actions. Narcissists are master hypocrites, and in inconsistency, they still need to keep their disguise on because, without them, their callous indifference would be on the show.

Their balanced disdain accounts for certain puzzling aspects narcissists have found, like no credentials, but a need to attack experts. Also, the evident confidence and self-assurance of the narcissist aren't genuine; their disdain towards their audience is the trustworthy source.

All this disdain leaves narcissists unwilling to discern emotionally between individuals and objects; that's why you always see narcissists enjoying things and using people. Commonly, people love people and use things. You may fall into the narcissist's scheme of things as an entity in their self-absorbed dreams to achieve unspoken objectives.

What may have prompted NPD to become a trend on the internet in recent years is that NPDs leave a trail of devastation in their wake. Even this trail was witnessed separately before the internet to connect victims to compare and share the stories of life. With internet access, patients come together, and NPD awareness is growing. One of the most interesting aspects found is how similar the perspectives of most victims are. Narcissistic violence is real; statistically, it is very pleasing among victims; it is not subjective mumbo jumbo. If it were simply a theory, considering the internet, NPD might never have gained any curiosity.

Signs and Symptoms of Narcissistic Personality Disorder

Until we speak about why it's important to stand back and first look at early warning signs and indications, to know why it's crucial but to defend yourself, you need to be able to read the terrain, notice it early. Analyzing risk is never as good as ignoring it altogether.

There are early symptoms in the process, and late in the relationship, we'll note down some of the more important signs and symptoms; it's rough again, so most of the time, you'll be sure of them because they fit the predictable trend of Love Bomb-Devalue and Dump.

Early Stages of Relationship-Love Bombing Symptoms:

- They present themselves as victims, essentially telling all the negative stories that happened to them. How people mistreated and exploited them, attracting sympathy for this approach and connecting you, even more, to help them, support them, and attempt and repair them.
- Too good to be real.
- In the first interactions, you communicate emotionally with them, and they mimic all about your personality characteristics, style, preferences and sound simple as if they are the nearest person to your character from day 1.
- You're the greatest thing that happens to them; nobody knows them, everybody has exploited them, and you're their salvation.
- The giant red flag that victims can look for is Parental Negligence or childhood violence; if they share it with you, particularly too soon, running for your life, it won't end well for you.
- They're going to love to blast you, raise you on a pedestal, essentially shower you with praises, and any compliment or feeling you give them will respond back

with more. They hook you up to their approval, love, adoration, and appreciation.

- They're really interested in you, telling you something about yourself, how was your day? They'll send you a lot of abnormal focus early on, start discussions first, speak to you for hours a day, win your confidence in this process, and get you addicted to the game.

- Unbearable mood swings, at one stage they're all lovely; at the other moment, they all erupt on you. You feel like you're moving on eggshells due to their erratic mood swings and they suck and rob your vitality alongside your esteem.

- They trigger trouble out of the blue as chaos brings fun to see how much you're able to handle and how much they can get away with; they create drama every day without any reason and then apologize, telling you they're overthinking. You don't know what to expect for the next second. It's their deception tactic to get you even more addicted to their game.

- They lavish you with all praise, respect, affection, compassion, concern, and they're like babies. They talk so early and want you to respond with the same stuff; that's the part they're trying to link you to their Empathy.

- Incredibly sexual at first encounter or chat, they'll try to hook you to their sexual game. If it doesn't work, they're going to be sensitive and lovely and going to insist that they remain with you.

Late Stages of Relationship-Devalue and Discard Symptoms:

- All love, adoration, respect, and care has demolished; they're cold and remote.

- Anything you do irritates them, even the jokes they used to chuckle at or the things you shared together.

- You're never enough to do anything; they keep dropping sarcasm per sentence.

- They get bored with you when they have no empathy and poor annoyance tolerance.

- You see their true face after 2-3 months that it was their performance, the person you believed they didn't live, it's an idea presented by them, their mask or façade drops off as acting takes a lot of energy.

- The love bombing continues to devalue.

- You feel like walking on eggshells, and you want attention, love, and care. They withhold their feelings; they withhold anything, you strive to find answers, but they don't give you any straightforward answers, only bland and cold answers, never establish contact first, lies floating over your mind. Meanwhile, they tell you they're lonely, and if you inquire for clarification, you're going to get nothing, you're getting tired of wasting focus, you don't know what to expect from this partnership, all the things going on in your mind you want some clarity, where they're giving you as little to hold in.

- When you want to lift an opinion or challenge the relationship to be a two-way street, ask them why they changed, or where the older person you once knew is, call them on their acts and lies, they refuse anything, exploit you with tactics.

Watch for these Four Characteristics

- **Gaslighting:** Denying anything you're saying, they're going to strike you today, and tomorrow they're going to convince you they haven't achieved it. They realize you're not going to leave everything simple. They're going to challenge you and your patience because they know you have a strong bond with them. They will make you question yourself and your hope.

- **Stone Walling:** You pose a question as to where their emotions are, she changes the subject and never responds, you ask a question about what they believe, they tell you they don't know, you never get a straightforward answer.

- **Silent Treatments:** Every time you call them on their behavior; this is the cruelest technique they can use; they disappear and give you the cold shoulder. They disappear for days, weeks, and even months without receiving any of your calls or texts; you don't know what happened. Through this tactic, they will avoid any liability for their acts; ignorance is their strongest weapon.

- **Projection:** Essentially, anytime you want to lift your opinion, you'll be punished for playing the victim card, convincing you that you're overthinking, even if you're confident that 100% did that. You end up explaining to them for the stuff you've never done, and they know deep down how much they're manipulating you; no matter what they're doing, they're still going to linger, and they've checked you early.

Do Narcissists Love? Love and Idealisation

Nope, they're idealizing. Let me tell you the distinction between affection and idealization.

Love: Willingness to empathize with a significant exchange of thoughts, concern, affection, love, value, and also a sincere feeling towards a person that involves emotions.

Idealization: A type of infatuation or fascination with a particular object or person; it does not contain any empathy.

The Narcissist: An adult with a body and a mind that lacks sensitivity and works on a four-year emotional basis is the average injured infant stuck in the adult body and mind that has never grown up mentally and has no idea what empathy entails from adolescence to chronic pain or violence.

The Development of Empathy: Empathy is the center of the personality; it begins to grow early in our adolescence, for example, for the child to represent the type of empathic individual that Empathy wants to gain in exchange, meaning affection, caring, consideration, respect, the importance of his or her parents. Empathy needs to be developed early in childhood; otherwise, if it does not develop, it will stagnate, and the infant will end up hollow as a shell.

WHAT MAKES A CHILD A CHILD? AND WHAT DIFFERS A GROWN-UP FROM A CHILD?

The most important thing that makes a child a child is its emotional level, whether you've found early on that the child loses emotion, for example, when it's developing, so it takes time. Likewise, a child attacks you unexpectedly and hits you in the face; you're injured. At the same moment, he laughs at his butt, and your parents tell you that it's just a kid that comes along, even if you're nuts, that's a lack of empathy; at the early stages of childhood, Empathy is underdeveloped. The grown-up has established their emotional level as they hit, for example, someone they're going to feel guilty for and lament that they later apologize for putting themselves in the other person's shoes.

What is the Narcissist Operating?

They begin with the idealization of a particular thing. Let's say an individual, once they idealize, they get a tunnel vision that becomes fascinated with that particular person because it's fresh and exciting. They still trust that they are in love with that person when they get high octane fuel from that person.

The distinction is that they don't love the person; they love the way that the person makes them feel for themselves. After some period, cracks tend to reappear as they have poor levels of boredom resistance; much like the average kid who gets overwhelmed with everything, the gap continues to emerge. Their internal fear is beginning to rise, and they are starting to doubt your worthiness, and you may not have been special, after all. And if you were the suffering that must have disappeared before now, that's going into their heads for someone new. Now they're beginning to groom new sources of supply when starting the Devaluation stage with you, which means they're trying to extract their emotions, resources, time, money, love from you.

Now, what's going to happen? When the tremendous amount of publicity has been attracted, the survivor continues to respond, not understanding what happened. They continue to ask the Narcissist questions and call them to action; they see this gesture as a huge danger to their safety. They begin to activate their defense mechanisms by exploiting a significant other to maintain their disguise or facade.

What is the Defence process? What are the Reactions?

For instance, you're calling them on their toxic behavior-they're trying to deny it entirely.

- You're asking for answers-they're not going to give you answers.
- You're hoping for a resolution—They're never going to give you closure.

- You call them on their actions-they're trying to change the subject or turn the blame on you and tell you that you're going nuts.

Bear in mind, the more the old source of supply or survivor asks, pleads, clings, the more control the narcissist feels, the more critical they feel. They have a weak ego, and the narcissist is behaving purely from the ego. Whatever the victim desires, they will withhold it because the victim has no more meaning in their minds because it has been replaced with a new enticing toy. They're not going to discard because any reaction from you would have made them the center of attention, and any reaction from you is still welcome; they feed on your reactions, be it a positive or an adverse reaction, so it makes them the center of attention. They see each person as objects; they cannot empathize with objects; any object is replaceable.

What the victims ought to remember? That it was never for them, it was just about the Narc, and they should never blame themselves for something they should accept it and step on because they were outstanding.

The Techniques Used to Manipulate the Victim as their Automatic Defensive Mechanism:

- **Gaslighting-Making**, you have questions about your sanity and vision.

- **Projection** of their feelings of inadequacy to you until their acts have been called upon.

- **Silent Treatments** – A form of passive violence used to neutralize the efforts to call them into toxic behavior, taking no blame or blame for it.

- **Stone Wall**-When you start looking for answers to change the subject or change the subject.

- **Emotional Withholds**, a type of retribution used by them if you keep them continuously calling for their toxic behavior, punishing you by denying caring, affection, attention, and treatment. Once the child loses the game, he or she refuses to play the game, or once you threaten the child with fact, he or she refuses to speak to you.

Is This Going to Happen Deliberately or Unintentionally?

This occurs as their unconscious reaction to the threat; this is their defense mechanism. A narcissist never plans to idealize another; it just happens. He never plans to devalue or dump anyone. It happens, though, because of frustration and their relentless hunger for supplies and all that's different, much as Adrenaline junkies searching for high or narcotics.

Easy Story To Enlighten Your Thoughts

For example, let's imagine a kid needs a pretty bad dog, a German Shepherd, and his mother buys him a dog, promising his mom that he's going to take care of the dog permanently and that he's going to embrace the dog forever.

The kid continues to idealize the dog because the dog is fresh and interesting; he's fascinated with the dog for a few weeks, months before he gets bored after he's bored and starts to devalue the dog because he's not fed empathy to the dog, not the emotional stage. He's leaving the dog to starve to death because he's bored, now what's going to happen? His mother takes over there to feed the dog and take responsibility for it.

Now the question is, would the child realize that he will idealize and undermine or discard the dog? Is that a plane? Not idealization and discarding happen as the baby gets bored; he would've never assumed the dog that the kid was fascinated with and would have dismissed it, nor would he ever have thought he would have glamorized the dog for a brief time.

Characteristics of Narcissist Personality

Grandiose Sense of Self-Importance

Grandiosity is the defining feature of narcissism. Rather than greed or pride, grandiosity is an excessive sense of dominance. Narcissists assume that they are exceptional or "special" and can only be recognized by such special individuals. What's worse, they're too smart for something standard or normal. They just want to interact and be affiliated with other high-level individuals, places, and stuff.

Narcissists also feel that they are better than anyone else and demand praise as such—even though they have done little to deserve it. They would also exaggerate or mislead clearly about their successes and skills. And when they talk about jobs or relationships, what you'll learn is how much they help, how amazing they are, and how grateful people are to have them in their lives. They're the undisputed star, and at best, everybody else is a bit of a player.

Lives in a Fantasy World that Supports their Delusions of Grandeur

Even though reality does not help their grandiose vision of themselves, narcissists exist in a fantasy universe powered by illusion, self-deception, and magical thinking. They're spinning self-glorifying dreams of infinite achievement, strength, brilliance, beauty, and perfect love that make them feel special and in control. These delusions shield them from feelings of inward emptiness and guilt, so they dismiss or rationalize the reality and views that contradict them. Anything that threatens to burst the dream bubble is greeted with intense defensiveness and even anger so that those surrounding the narcissist learn to proceed cautiously around their ignorance of the truth.

Needs Constant Praise and Admiration

A narcissist's feeling of entitlement is like a balloon that is steadily losing air without a constant supply of applause and validation to keep it inflated. Occasional compliments are not enough. Narcissists need daily fuel for their ego, so they associate themselves with others who can accept their obsessive craving for approval. These ties are rather one-sided. It's about what the admirer will do to the narcissist, and not the other way around. And if the admirer's devotion and praise are either disrupted or reduced, the narcissist sees it as a betrayal.

Sense of Entitlement

Since they believe themselves superior, narcissists perceive preferential consideration as their due. They really think they should get whatever they want. They still want the people around them to satisfy their single wish and whim immediately. This is their only meaning. If you're not expecting and satisfying their every desire, then you're worthless. And if you're worried about undermining their will or "selfishly" hoping for something in return, brace yourself for aggression, anger, or a cold shoulder.

Exploits Others Without Guilt or Shame

Narcissists never cultivate the capacity to connect with other people's feelings—to put themselves in other people's shoes. Or other words, they lack sympathy. In certain ways, they see people in their lives as objects—to fulfill their needs. As a result, they do not think twice about taking advantage of others to reach their goals. Perhaps this behavioral manipulation is intentional, but sometimes it is just evident. Narcissists don't care about how their actions influence people. Even if you find that out, they're probably not really going to get it. The only thing they can comprehend is their own needs.

Frequently Demeans, Intimidates, Bullies, or Belittles Others

Narcissists feel threatened if they meet someone who seems to have what they lack—especially those who are optimistic and famous. They're often challenged by people who don't crow or question them in any way. Their defense mechanism is disdain. The only way to neutralize the hazard and shore up their sluggish ego is to tear those people down. They can do so in a patronizing or insensitive manner as if to prove how little the other person matters to them. Or they can strike with slurs, name-calling, abuse, and threats to push the other person back into line.

Reasoning with a Narcissist

To understand them, you need to understand their logic. Narcissists act in the manner they do since their unique mode of logic inspires them, motivates them, and compels them. The selfish and narcissistic logic was inseparable. They can't step in anyone else's shoes; they can't see beyond their narcissistic square. They're like a programming program, inexorable, relentless, free of extraneous concerns.

Initially, this narcissistic argument is difficult to distinguish (because it is so new to us). Yet, it is pretty easy to understand when you see that it is focused entirely on thoughts and feelings. Thoughts and feelings solely drive the narcissists. This means that when they want something, they can't access logic. But there's something to that; the feelings and emotions they use to negotiate their goals just include their own emotions and feelings. Your emotions are never heard; they are meaningless, either because you don't exist as a human or because you are considered dumb. When you assert your thoughts and needs, you're going to be more complicated to block out. If they could understand the feelings, they could not be narcissists in the very first place. You're dealing with a creature who has never known about someone else's emotions before.

If a manipulative argument is presented, the narcissist cannot understand the reasoning and cannot understand the reality of the emotions and needs. Objective reasoning or the desires and emotions are unreasonably and illogical to the narcissist. Reasoning from logical reasoning or justifying your own desires seems stupid and unwise to the narcissist because something the narcissist does instantly understand is inherently stupid, and the narcissist often thinks like you are attempting to trick them by using your flawed, incomprehensible logic or prioritizing your own selfish needs. The more you try, the more unwise and foolish you look, or the more you appear to want to defraud them, the more you dig your own grave when you do that. Trying to speak sense to a narcissist makes you seem dumb or seem to be conniving to them. The only reasoning that doesn't seem stupid; the only thing they should trust is how they feel. It's a practical reality of how they feel is logical. Therefore, there can never be a bridge of awareness between you and the narcissist.

Those who can know the language of the narcissist's feelings will be able to trick the narcissist out of their residence and household. So when it comes to important problems of life, typically those that include bargaining between their emotions and the sufferings and inconveniences that they bring others, the narcissist can argue purely and exclusively about what they desire, never for what makes sense logically or if it impacts others. Narcissistic reasoning is locked inside, circular, and self-consistent by self-referencing. They make full sense to themselves but only to themselves, not even to other narcissists), and use the idiosyncratic vocabulary of their impulses and sheer subjectivity. Anything that sounds like a second language to them, and there are no shared meanings because they can't understand 'outside things.' For instance, you don't exist as an individual, and so neither will your needs (that proposition is intellectually coherent, as long as you don't actually exist).

Moreover, no one else lives anymore, but there is no objectivity, either the lack of object constancy, the philosophy of mind). That's why the narcissist can't grasp how you're mad or that this or that is unjust to anyone. The narcissists are natural solipsists. If there was no tree in the forest and the narcissist was not present, there was no sound. It didn't collapse, though, and the forest didn't exist either.

So, for example, you're in a relationship with a narcissist, and you're always saving up for a new home, the narcissist is unexpectedly buying a red luxury car, you're never going to end up having the new home. Trying to talk about the goals of a race car and a new home would irritate the narcissist. The harder you try, the less you make sense of the narcissist. The sports car looked amazing, and that's why it was bought instantly. Period. Period. The idea of a new home doesn't feel perfect. Talking about saving up for a new house doesn't make much sense and is dumb; this sort of stupid talk bothers the narcissist. You bother the narcissist with your dumb logic and selfish desires and emotions. The more you continue, the more irritated the narcissist gets because you don't make much sense; just bragging about the joy of a new car makes any sense. Criticizing sports cars leads the narcissist to devalue you, to mock you further to devalue you further. This is how the friendship began.

And that's why, when you and the narcissist enjoy mutual pleasures or views, the narcissist is such a barrel of fun. Still, when struggling with conflicts, the narcissist is impossible. The trick to understanding is that the narcissist goes for something that makes them feel good but avoids something that doesn't or makes them feel depressed. When they're fine, they're perfect; when they're bad, they're terrible.

What Causes a Person to Become a Narcissist?

Narcissistic Personality Traits are a by-product of unique childhood family environments. Both children want the consent and affection of their parents. Kids adapt to their homes, and perhaps the most effective and rational adaptation to such home conditions is to become a narcissist.

Below are several typical scenarios that may make children narcissistic.

Scenario 1—Narcissistic Parent Ideals

In this case, the infant is born in a home that is very competitive and awards just high achievement. One or two of the parents are an exhibitionist narcissist. The motto of the family is If you can't be the best, why bother?

When you're first in the competition to win the science fair or the star at the school presentation, you're full of recognition and focus. You're a failure because you don't. All in the family is meant to be special and to show that again and again. No matter how much you do, the burden is never gone.

Kids in these households don't feel permanently loved. It's hard for them to love something for their own sake because it confers status. Instead of being encouraged by their parents to discover what they want and wish to do more, they only earn systems with high achievement. Their parents are not involved in their children's "real selves," they are most interested in how their children will make the family look fine. They would like to be able to feel good to their neighbors: "Look what my child did!"

Kids who grow up in households like this feel safe and worthwhile because they are successful and accepted as the 'best.' The conditional affection of their youth and the overvaluation of high status and achievement in their home set in motion a lifelong cycle of attainment of success and confusion with satisfaction.

Scenario 2: The Narcissistic Parent Devaluation

In this case, there is a very authoritative and devaluing adult who is constantly bringing the kid down. The parent is usually irritable, readily angry, and has unrealistically high aspirations. If there are two or more twins, the parent may praise one and devalue the other. The "good one will easily become the "bad one, and suddenly a new sibling is raised. Nobody in the family feels safe, and they all spend their time attempting to quiet the explosive Manipulative mom.

The other parent is also viewed just like an infant and often belittled. When he or she argues with the narcissistic parent, the two of them are devalued. Kids who grow up in these homes are furious, ashamed, and insufficient. They are likely to respond in a few different ways to their childhood condition.

The Vanquished Child: A few of these children just give up and embrace defeat. In their teenage years, after decades of being told that they are useless, they may descend into self-hating shame-based depression. Then to relieve their inner guilt, they may attempt to lose themselves in impetuous, addictive behavior. Some of them become alcoholics and opioid addicts; others waste their days on the Phone. They never reach their ability because they were told they had none.

The Rebel Child:

These children openly ignore the message of their parents that they are "losers." Instead, they spend their lives seeking to prove to themselves the world and the devaluing parent that they are special and that their parents are incorrect. They're seeking success in whatever direction they can. Proving that they are unique becomes a lifetime task, while beneath, there is still a stern inner voice condemning any mistake—no matter how slight.

The Wretched Child:

These children grow up frustrated with the devaluing mom. Anyone who reminds them of their parents in any way becomes the object of their wrath. Even they themselves turn poisonous or malignant narcissists. It's not enough for them to do that; they have to kill as well.

Scenario 3: " The Golden Child"

These parents are typically close-up narcissists who are awkward in the spotlight. Instead, they brag about their very talented boy. Often the kid is very creative and deserves attention, but even these parents take it to insane lengths. This form of extreme idealization of an infant as flawless and unique will contribute to a superficial adaptation of the child in later life.

The Consequences of Reciprocal vs. Unconditional Love

All deserve to be treated realistically and to be loved unconditionally. If children assume that their parents respect them simply because they are unique, this may add to the underlying vulnerability. No one's going to win all the way. No one in any way is better than anyone else. Children who are idealized by a parent will continue to assume that they are lovable only because they are flawless and deserving of idealization.

Knowledge of the Mistakes and the Guilt

When parents idealize their offspring, they can be afraid to find the defects in themselves. This will lead them to try to aspire for excellence and to show that they are beautiful and capable of idealization.

Shocked Production of the True Self

In this phase, children can lose contact with their true selves and real likes and dislikes. Instead of discovering who they actually are and where their true passions and strengths lie, they can get off track and waste their time only doing stuff that they're already good at, and they hope their parents can get their approval.

The result: Much more parental idealization can lead to an imbalanced view of the self. When this happens, the kid sees all defects as intolerable and strives to be treated as flawless. It's a short hop, a skip, and a jump from here to the full-blown narcissism.

Scenario 4: Admirer of the Exhibitionist

Some kids end up in a narcissistic family where there is an airhead narcissist parent who presents them with affection and recognition as long as they respect and remain subservient to their parents. These children are taught selfish ideals but are prohibited from allowing themselves to be appreciated. Instead, their position in the family is to worship the superiority of their authoritarian parent uncritically without ever attempting to match or transcend the parent's achievement.

This is a perfect way to build Cover or Closet Narcissists. The children understand that they will gain narcissistic supplies—attention and praise—for not openly interfering with the narcissistic parent and that these supplies will be withdrawn and devalued if they openly attempt to be regarded as unique. All their importance in the family comes from serving as a boost to the Exhibitionist parent's ego.

In adulthood, these children feel too humiliated and insecure about being secure in the spotlight, but their narcissism and self-esteem problems are less apparent to someone who may not know them well. May may well adjust to this task and lead fruitful lives in a job that includes helping a highly accomplished exhibitionist narcissist, whom they respect.

How Does a Narcissist Behave?

Narcissists are very selective of the vocabulary they use, and they try to use expressions that support their diabolical aims and raise their ego. Sometimes when their words are directed at others, they are meant to annoy and disturb their prey. They're trying to say stuff like you're too sensitive" or you've misunderstood me" to make you believe that your answer to them is unjustified and that you ought to project your own personal problems.

Or maybe they'll play their own classic "I hate drama" card as tensions escalate to suggest that you and not them are the root of nonsense when in fact, they're behind it. Narcissists are sure to have a handful of those damaging words that they enjoy, so look out for this characteristic as a strong indication that you're dealing with one.

Snipe, They're Directing/Aiming at You

You should be careful of someone who always tries to bring others down (both in their faces and behind their backs). Those dumb remarks are subtle, but they are packed with negativity. While they may not sound like anything in isolation, when they arise on a daily basis, they may be extremely harmful to the person they are being targeted at.

It's Still the Blame of Someone Else

A narcissist never feels that they've done wrong (they're gods). If someone is to blame in their eyes, they're still someone else. To accept remorse would be like an arrow in the center of a narcissist's ego, so they would attempt to transfer blame to others around them. But they blame the guy, his confounding and exhausting allegation that casts doubt in their minds and makes them feel insecure about their acts.

They're Not Afraid to Use Lies to Get their Way

They're going to take the facts, twist it, and insist that you're mistaken anytime you want and tell it like it was. They're going to make you doubt yourself. They're going to drive you crazy, your memory, and your convictions by forcing a distorted sense of truth upon you. And if you pretend to have witnesses, they will deny its existence or accuse you of making it seem foolish and devilish.

They've got Jekyll & Hyde Identities

A narcissist may be friendly and polite when he or she needs to be; indeed, this is also how they pursue friendship and more with their victims. They can only act in such a way, though when it is necessary, and the act is easily dropped when someone is hooked or enmeshed.

Why a Narcissist Acts the Way they Do?

Narcissus can be charming, charismatic, seductive, thrilling, and entertaining. They can also behave exploitatively, arrogantly, fiercely, coldly, competitively, selfishly, shamefully, cruelly, and vindictively. You could fall in love with their charming side and be devastated by their dark side. It may be baffling, but it all makes sense to consider what drives them. This knowledge saves you from their games, propaganda, and exploitation.

Narcissists have a self that is impaired or undeveloped. They think and behave differently than other people. The level of narcissism varies. Other individuals show more symptoms of more extreme lavishness, and other narcissists have less, milder symptoms. Consequently, the above discussion does not extend to all narcissists to the same degree.

Narcism Vulnerability

Despite possessing obviously powerful attitudes, narcissists are actually fragile. Psychotherapists view them as "fragile." They suffer from extreme loneliness, emptiness, powerlessness, and loss of purpose. Because of their intense weakness, they want the power to watchfully monitor their world, the people around them, and their emotions. Displays of fragile emotions such as anxiety, guilt, or sorrow, are unacceptable indicators of vulnerability in both themselves and others. Their protection mechanism protects them, but it harms others, particularly when they feel the most unsafe.

Narcissistic Disgrace

There is a poisonous embarrassment under their facade, and they could be unaware. The guilt helps narcissists feel unsafe and inadequate—vulnerable emotions that they must suppress to themselves and others. That's one factor they can't bear critique, accountability, dissension, or derogatory reviews, even though it's supposed to be positive. Instead, they are demanding unconditional, constructive treatment from others.

Awesomeness

Their secret guilt is due to their braggadocio and self-aggrandizement. They try to persuade themselves and others that they shine, that they are uniquely exceptional and the best, the brightest, the wealthiest, the most beautiful, and the most talented. This is also why narcissists gravitate towards celebrities and high-ranking individuals, colleges, corporations, and other organizations. Being among the strongest convinces them that they're better than most, but psychologically, they're not so confident.

Failure of Empathy

The capacity of narcissists to respond emotionally and communicate sufficient treatment and concern is greatly diminished. (See "Can a Narcissist Love?.") Without sympathy, narcissists can be greedy, hurtful, and cold when it doesn't serve them to be charming or cooperative. Relationships are transactional to them. Rather than listening to emotions, they are interested in fulfilling their needs—sometimes, even though it involves manipulating others, stealing, misleading, or violating the rule. While they may experience joy and desire at the early stages of a relationship, this is not loving but lust. They're known for their game-play. Their lack of sympathy often inspires them to feel the pain that they cause people, while their social-emotional intellect gives them the edge to control and abuse others to fulfill their needs.

Vacuity

Narcissists lack a positive, emotional connection to themselves, making it impossible for them to communicate emotionally with others. Their undeveloped self-resources and lack of inner resources require them to be dependent on others for affirmation. Despite their self-indulgence, they yearn for recognition and endless admiration. Since their sense of worth is influenced by what people think about them, they want to influence what others think they feel better about themselves. They use partnerships for self-enhancement and for their "narcissistic supply." But because of their inner emptiness, they are never fulfilled. Like the vampires who are dead inside, the narcissists manipulate and drain those around them.

Lack of Boundary

Mythological Narcissus fell in love with his own portrait, mirrored in a pool of water. At first, he didn't know it was himself. Narcissists metaphorically represent this. The inner emptiness, guilt, and undeveloped selves of the narcissists make them unaware of their limits. They can not experience other people as distinct entities, but as two-dimensional extensions of themselves, without emotions, because narcissists cannot empathize. Some people live solely to satisfy their needs. This is why narcissists are narcissistic and indifferent to their effect on others, particularly though they are cruel.

Narcissism Defenses

It is the defensive mechanisms used by narcissists to shield their insecurity that make relations with narcissists so challenging. The typical defenses they use are superiority and disrespect, denial, projection, hostility, and jealousy.

Types of Narcissists

Narcissism is multi-faceted and comes in a variety of forms. Narcissists can employ a number of strategies and protections to make you unsafe and ensuring that their rank and needs are met. It's easy to be puzzled, but it's important to recognize and spot what kind of narcissist you're dealing with. Recently two research groups have identified a shared function.

The Grandiose Narcissist

While there are various kinds and degrees of narcissism, for years, literature has concentrated mostly on the familiar—exhibitionist narcissists that pursue the limelight. There are the magnificent grandiose narcissists that are prominent figures and are visible in films. They are listed in the Diagnostic Statistical Manual of Psychiatric Disorders (DSM) under narcissistic personality disorder (NPD).

We should all spot such charming, thought-provoking extroverts whose arrogance and boldness are at times obnoxious and shameless. They are self-absorbed, justified, callous, exploitative, totalitarian, and violent. Any of them are sexually violent. These unsympathetic, narcissistic narcissists think so well about themselves but spare no contempt for anyone.

Helped by their extraversion, they report high self-esteem and happiness with their lives despite the suffering of others. Since they outwardly desire acclaim, publicity, and dominance, grandiose narcissism is outsourced. Even in love, they're hunting for strength by playing sports. Many sustain partnerships, considering the lack of affection and unhappiness of their spouses, who are quickly seduced by their charm and boldness.

The Vulnerable Narcissist

Little identified are insecure narcissists (also referred to as underground narcissists, closets, or introverted narcissists). Like their grandiose kinsmen, they are self-absorbed, justified, exploitative, unsympathetic, manipulative, and violent, but they are so fearful of scrutiny that they shy away from scrutiny. Individuals in both forms of narcissism also lack autonomy, have imposter syndrome, a poor sense of self, are self-alienated, and unable to regulate their setting. However, vulnerable narcissists perceive these things to a far larger degree.

Unlike grandiose narcissists, rather than feeling secure and self-satisfied, insecure narcissists are unsure and dissatisfied with their lives. They're feeling more pain, fear, remorse, sadness, hypersensitivity, and embarrassment. They are in disagreement, maintaining both inflated and pessimistic irrational expectations of themselves—the latter that they place on other people, their lives, as well as the future. Their negative feelings represent a bitter neurotic aversion to personal development. They need affirmation of their grandiose self-image and are extremely defensive when perceived feedback causes a poor perception of themselves.

They ignore meaningful relationships, unlike extroverted narcissists. Instead of boldly dominating others, they are threat-oriented and distrustful. Their form of attachment is more avoidable and nervous. They detach from others with violent shame and anger, internalizing their narcissism. Empathetic co-dependents feel compassionate and try to spare them from their suffering, but end up self-sacrificing and feeling responsible for them.

The Communal Narcissist

Far more challenging to classify is the third form of narcissist named only recently—communal narcissists. They admire comfort, compassion, and elegance. They see themselves and want others to see it as the most reliable and friendly atmosphere, and they seek to accomplish this through kindness and kindness. They're going out like a grandiose narcissist. But while the grandiloquent narcissist wants to be seen as the smartest and most powerful, the communal narcissist wants to be seen as the most gifted and helpful. The vain selflessness of communal narcissists is no less selfish than that of a grandiose narcissist. They both share common motivations for grandiosity, esteem, entitlement, and strength, though each employs different activities to accomplish them. It's a bigger plunge as their hypocrisy is revealed.

The Malign Narcissist

Malignant narcissists are known to be at the end of the spectrum of narcissism because of their brutality and aggressiveness. They're cynical, immoral, and sadistic. They take joy in causing confusion and dragging people down. These narcissists are not inherently grandiose, extroverted, or neurotic, but they are closely linked to psychiatry, the dark triad, and anti-social personality disorder.

Fluctuating States of Ego

If you have a hard time recognizing which sort of narcissist you're working with, that could be because grandiose narcissists are oscillating between states of grandiosity and weakness. For example, grandiose narcissists can exhibit insecurity and emotionality (usually anger) when their performance is reversed or their self-conception is under threat. More fantastic grandiosity suggests greater uncertainty and the possibility of variability. There is no proof that vulnerable narcissists display excellence.

The Search for the Core of Narcissism

Recent studies have begun to distinguish a singular, unifying characteristic between narcissists. Researchers looked at narcissism by examining distinct personality characteristics. Two recent models have emerged: one based on individuality and the other on an open, transactional leadership style.

The Trifurcated Model

The Trifurcated Model of Narcissism reveals that narcissism relies on three personality traits: agentic extraversion, discomfort, and neuroticism. (Agentic extraverts are authoritative and bold go-getters who occupy positions of acclaim, success, and leadership.) Of the Big Five personality characteristics, disabling is the only one common to all styles. The paradigm sheds light on the nature of narcissism as emotional antagonism, shared by grandiose and fragile narcissists both. It is characterized by coercion, aggression, entitlement, callousness, and rage (Kaufman et al., 2020). Vulnerable and majestic narcissists express antagonism differently. The former is more aggressive while distrustful; the latter are more immodest and powerful.

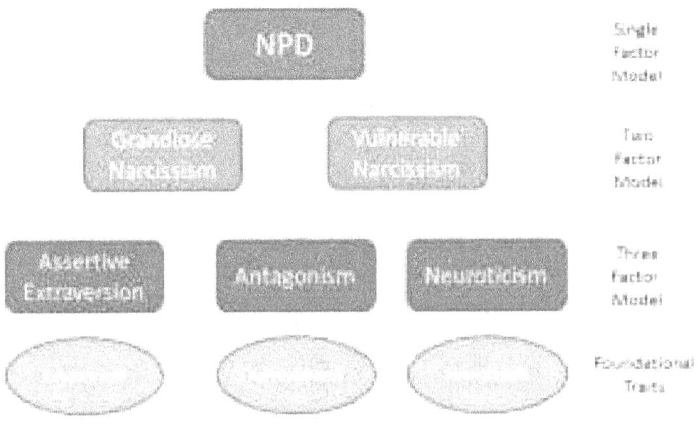

The Spectrum Model

The Narcissism Continuum Model (NSM) developed by Kerzan and Herlache (2017) conceives of narcissism as occurring on a spectrum from grandiose to fragile. It illustrates how the NPD differs in magnitude and how the traits present themselves. The model indicates that all forms of narcissists have a similar psychological center of self-importance. Narcissists believe that they and their interests are unique and that they take priority over those of others. This essence consists of greed, self-involvement, and entitlement. In reality, entitlement is reported to be the most toxic factor in relationships.

Narcissism Spectrum Model

Entitled Self-Importance

Grandiose Narcissists   Vulnerable Narcissists

The multiple identities of narcissists convey varying qualities at different moments; this model captures a complex, systematic study that is more reflective of real life. The greater the grandeur of an individual, the less fragile they are and vice versa. More privilege and risk-taking raise professional and emotional challenges. The greater the weakness, the more away (, the lower) is their grandiosity.

Takeaways

In brief, narcissism occurs on a continuum ranging from dominant and extroverted to introverted and neurotic. The central characteristics of narcissism are antagonism, self-importance, and entitlement, rendering narcissists unfavorable, uncooperative spouses, and work colleagues. Since other forms of personality may be antagonistic, I favor the Continuum Paradigm, which defines self-important superiority as the center of narcissism, separating it from sociopathy and paranoid personality disorder, among others.

Grandiose narcissists are presenting a mixed bag. Although they feel and work differently than vulnerable narcissists and can be socially active when they want, their antagonism and entitlement causes issues and endangers relationships. When they are taking part in counseling, they should focus on their antagonism and privilege.

On the other hand, vulnerable narcissists require assistance in controlling their attitudes, moods, and feelings. They mimic individuals with borderline personality disorder and may benefit from dialectical behavioral treatment that is effective in mitigating antagonism. Schema-focused psychotherapy and cognitive behavioral therapy are effective for all styles of minimizing guilt and anger.

Whatever sort of narcissist you care for, your friendship is hurtful. Instead of fulfilling your desires, you are weakened and drained by frequent criticism, callousness, aggression, requests, and legitimate aspirations. Don't waste your time trying to impress or change a narcissist. Instead, launch the healing to restore your self-esteem and autonomy and make you more resilient whether you stay or go. While you are undecided, take some person psychotherapy and use the Narcissist Dealing Methods to assess the relationship's prognosis.

PART 2: HANDLING THE NARCISSIST

Identifying a Narcissist

People with Narcissistic Personality Disorder are incredibly difficult to spot. And trained psychologists who have no first-hand experience (as a victim) are easily tricked. One of the world's foremost rehabilitation professionals, he was himself a working psychologist before he fell victim to a sexual narcissistic relationship – and his world turned upside down. But how on earth can anyone decide whether or not they have a narcopath on their hands?

Machiavelli

All successful con artists need brilliant tricks to get away from their audacious deceptions, and the narcopath is no different. They will be proud of their unscrupulous and treacherous ways of demanding stage appearances by an accomplished performer, but the narcissist has been honing his acting abilities since early childhood. Although others are never in the ranks, the unfortunate fact is that many are professionals and carry out their positions with distinction – literally. They are to all intents and purposes, the very cornerstone of society-in commissions, an active member of the Church, with occupations as distinguished as they can be.

Look Tough Then look at it again

Although there are a variety of indications where, if you are cynical enough to press hard, you should be given a fair hint, cunning and deceptive as they can be, these are the red flags I'm looking for.

Loving Bombarding

Narcissists know that they have to get you hooked and addicted before they continue to extract their manipulative supplies from you. They're doing this with love-bombing. Expect lots of compliments, daily texts, and messages of undying affection and desire. Right from the get-go, they intend to manipulate the mind on an hourly basis. This plays a secondary role – the growth of your confidence in someone else. Messages of sound very familiar and not actually personalized directly to you – and that's because they're not real or original, but they're copied from movies, books, and the like. Don't forget; Narc's simply don't have the same feelings as normal-range people do because they can't experience affection. So you're being courted by the same charade that's their whole life.

The Mirror

By mirroring, narcissists put themselves as the soul mate. Anticipate a lot of in-depth questions in the early days when they get to know you. Getting to know one-other is common in a relationship, but with a narcissist, it's more like research, and it's really one-sided. They're not going to give it away until you've shown it first. Then they will claim to enjoy all the same stuff as you do – activities, past-times, games, passions, music, food, places to visit, drinks, etc.

A lot of Elegance

They know how to win people over easily, and they're going to come off really charming – but for those people who count.' Expect the vicary to be handled very differently from the garbage collector. The charisma, though, is fake – something that their "false self" uses to give the appearance of a decent person, a cornerstone of civilization. Their romantic partners are only really seeing their charming sides in public – in secret, giving up hope now.

Great Ego

This is the characteristic of an accessible narcissist – brash, full of his own successes, disrespectful of others, dismissive of mistakes, unaccountable for his cock-ups, vane, and excessively preoccupied with his picture. Many would be able to see politicians and actors slipping into these stereotypes. But beware, while this may be a crucial gift to open-minded narcissists, many other types of narcissists do not suit this template. Also, with the hidden ones, though, once you get to know them personally, you're going to have this intense sense that in their lives, it's all about them.

Nice Listener

Don't mistake this one for the warm and kind type of listening and empathizing – the narcissist's way of listening is more thoughtful to research. In the beginning, narcos are searching for ways to get their hooks into you, indications of vulnerability, a hint of the narcissistic fuel tank that you serve, what makes you tick, etc.

Fast to Intimacy

The standard spectrum of individuals give time for their feelings to grow – and these emotions come naturally. Less so for the narcissist, who actually cannot sense the intimacy of feelings. They're on a supply-derived mission, and they're very irritated with normal-range objectives taking their time.

Sexually Excessively

Although they might not be willing to experience affection, sexual conquest is a validation and thus a selfish source of drugs. So expect them to be sexual until your degree of intimacy is properly built.

A lot of Crazies

Narcs are leaving a trail of devastation in their tracks. Yet they themselves cannot be kept responsible for this state of affairs – so it must be their victims, right? Look out for the narco to dismiss their exes and so on as nuts or to make a screw loose. And they're always abusive – they're masters of transferring their own flaws into their victims.

High Mood

Although they may be trying to impress you and behave themselves accordingly, they never seem to have a rather haughty attitude – particularly to people like restaurant waiters. Look for self-importance, pomposity, rudeness, and self-improvement.

Controlling the Situation

They have to monitor circumstances, particularly their spouse and children, household finances, social responsibilities, family plans. Just those that they can confidently monitor are allowed to join their core group of friends. Those who demonstrate critical thinking and independent thinking are kept at a distance.

Lack of Genuine Apology

Narcopaths are struggling to repent, really about something. They simply can't be mistaken – admitting that it dents their sense of a perfect "false self." They either freeze, change the subject, or else dodge, or mumble an apology followed by a "but... ".

You're working on Eggshells

In normal friendships and partnerships, the connection should be solid enough to feel secure that you could disagree or tell them any truths about your home. For a narcopath, you can sense an unwritten law and intestine sensation where you don't question them. Ever ever. What's more, they can also smell the mood that they're furious and on the brink of the blast, so you have to step cautiously.

Core of Focus

Narcopaths enjoy being the focus of attention and hate being cared about by someone else-especially members of the same sex. Their favorite subject of discussion is, you guessed it yourself. They're going to aspire to sit in the middle of a huge dining table, and they're going to be the first to dance on the chairs, they're going to expect high spirits at events.

Sycophant

Narcs enjoy being considered to be synonymous with higher-intellectual individuals – but perversely hate being eclipsed by them. They are especially suspicious of someone who could be found more beautiful than they are.

Lack of Continuity of Object

Like a chameleon, narcos can be customized to better shine based on the organization or the condition they are in. Invariably, behind closed doors, they would treat their closest and dearest accordingly. So whether it's their political affiliation, hobbies, preferences, favorite food, or hue – expect things to change any time the wind blows.

Achievement by Robbers

Their mixture of laziness and entitlement, and given the charade of fake selves, you will find that they are great at declaring the hard work and success of others as theirs. Those are the managers who are hard taskmasters to their subordinates while they are too busy brown-nosing their elders and winding and dining customers to roll their sleeves. Those are the partners who miss domestic tasks when they're too busy somewhere else, somewhere else. There are the couples who bum all day and trust the other half of them to get the bacon around.

Above the Rule of Law

Their lack of sympathy for people spreads to a broader culture – no one else. Connect to that their propensity for risk, their pathological lies, and their sense of superiority, and you can understand why an estimated 25 percent of the prison population has NPD.

100 Ways to Know if You are a Victim of Narcissist Abuse

1. You've got the gut sense that something is wrong, that there is stuff you don't know about.

2. You hear contradictory stories about them that don't make any sense.

3. You're going to trap them in lies, like lies that wouldn't make much sense to say.

4. You think them nice to the people you hear them talk ill of when they're not around.

5. Not only are they angry over small things, including things that don't sound rational or make sense. You can't imagine that anybody's going to get mad over that stuff, even though they're just having a bad day. The rage is coming out of nowhere.

6. You find yourself doing something you've never done in the past or experiencing things in reaction to a partner's actions that you've never felt in comparable circumstances with others or in the past.

7. You're always being accused of stealing.

8. When you try to involve them in a discussion about something that happened in a relationship that you find unjust or hurtful, the conversation turns into nonsense, and they end up turning it around on you and accusing you of initiating an argument.

9. One upon a time, the love-bombing was over the top, and you thought you had found a soulmate.

10. Their acts do not reflect the terms they utter much of the time.

11. They're going from loving you to hating you immediately, or they're suddenly going to say you don't exist.

12. They barely show regret; even if they do, they go back to doing the same stuff they said they were guilty of.

13. You're separated from the ones you care about most.

14. They talk poorly about people or things you care about, and they threaten you to stop people or things like that.

15. They stay in close touch with you while the two of you are not together, and they clothe it as being concerned. "

16. They're looking for hidden nuances in what you've said, and they're taking neutral stuff as critique.

17. They always change plans for you then want you to change yours when the hat drops.

18. You see them manipulating knowledge, only letting out enough and/or saying something to people to get what they want.

19. You find yourself wary of strangers you've never met because of what you've been taught about.

20. They do terrible stuff, but somehow they have an excuse for it.

21. You're getting nervous when you're with them, uncertain of how they're going to respond.

22. They talk to people they always say they can't get up and look like you're mad when you bring it up.

23. You find yourself protecting them or shielding their horrible acts from others.

24. You don't want to call their actions manipulative, or maybe it doesn't feel like being exploited – it just sounds so overwhelming.

25. When they go, you're desperate to miss them and don't understand why.

26. You sound like you have a special bond with them.

27. They're going to make you be in regular touch with them while you're out with your friends.

28. They've got a phone full of people they've been in relationships with in the past or people they've just met, but don't want you to have friends at all, especially the opposite sex.

29. You can't concentrate on something except being obsessed with trying to figure out the friendship.

30. You find yourself trying to pick between pushing them on petty lies or letting it go.

31. Some of the lies they're telling are so vast, and they encompass having completely separate lives and making people for themselves who don't exist.

32. You feel like you're losing your mind.

33. They bait you to respond and then use your response to make you feel as though you are to blame for the death of the relationship or as if you deserve to be handled.

34. They're using stuff that you told them against you, and they're saying other people things that you told them confidently.

35. You're going to be mentally ill with no clarification.

36. You lost your self-esteem.

37. You have lost your employment, financial status, or other simple means of survival, or ways of sustaining yourself.

38. They pushed you to do stuff you didn't want to do.

39. They've made threats to hurt you physically or mentally.

40. People have turned against you in your life because of your friendship.

41. They enabled you to indulge in deviant conduct and then threatened to use it against you.

42. You're going to go, but you can't stop talking to them.

43. You want them to leave you alone; however, you want them to get in touch with you.

44. They're intruding on your privacy.

45. They waste a long time in the shower, making excuses for what they're doing there.

46. You start disassociating or withdrawing.

47. You still know like something is wrong.

48. You're sexually assaulted, so you're considered too emotional.

49. You're always on the verge, and there's no rhyme or explanation that a good night will instantly change everything that has been said. It'll set them off instinctively, and a nice night with them would suddenly turn into a nightmare. Then they pretend that it never happened, not apologizing for their actions.

51. Anything, but you don't have to do the same thing.

52. You catch yourself apologizing, even if you're not exactly what you've done anything.

53. You also feel as if they clash with you or are jealous of you and try to undermine you.

54. You always feel like they see you smiling because they're not the source; they want to do something to spoil it. Holidays, birthdays, and special days always end with pain.

55. You're full of questions, and you never get any answers.

56. Sometimes, you're not able to pick what you want to watch while they're present because when you are, they're mocked or punished.

57. They push you to hang out with their mates. However, they can place you in a double bond by accusing you of being unfriendly if you don't communicate enough with your friends or flirting if you interact "too much with them.

58. They also have cheating or psychotic exes who have treated them poorly in the past to justify why they are behaving so badly towards you today, along with several other reasons. More possibly, they produced the "crazy ex, who was actually manipulated and not psychotic.

59. They often compare you to past exes, preferably at first. Deeper in the relationship, in order to make you feel unsafe, they can continue to associate you unfavorably with exes in order to influence your actions and get you to do something or not do something. "My ex has never done that or "My ex has always done that..."

60. You often feel like your partner is two different people, and you're constantly trying to figure out which one is the "real" one.

61. Their reaction to being questioned is smug indignation, not regret.

62. They respond with frustration when they feel that you've kept something secret from them or haven't involved them in a decision or operation.

63. They deliberately keep secret some of their actions and emotions.

64. You are not permitted to have regular human responses or feelings to typical events.

65. Usually, their reaction to your feelings is to quit or place the attention back on themselves.

66. When they feel like you've wronged them – whether you have it or not – they're going to find a way to blame you for it.

67. They're behaving one way in public and another way in private because you're the only one there.

68. You find justifications for their actions, such as, "He's just a passionate person," or He's been hurt so much in the past," or He's just having a bad day."

69. Your friends and family told you that you should get away from him or her or that you're not the same person you used to be.

70. You're always looking forward to the "good old days" that prevailed when you first met your girlfriend.

71. Often, you're terrified of your mate.

72. Often, you feel really bad, and sometimes you don't even know why.

73. Your companion is a chronic liar.

74. Your companion is excellent at making his or herself a suspect, and you've discovered that he or she would also cheat you to do so.

75. Your wife has threatened to kill you or yourself if you leave your relationship.

76. Your wife has threatened to have the police involved if you left the relationship or have made any direct threats to your life or well-being if you said you would leave.

77. Your wife is trying to dictate how you look, where you go, or how you spend your time.

78. They're quitting the relationship every time they don't get the answer they expect, but they're still coming back because every time you feel like you have to give up more and more of yourself if you want them to stop doing that. You know this means that, for example, you have to avoid telling them about those topics.

79. When you show feelings or weep, often they have almost no emotion at all or even appear irritated or sometimes entertained by your discomfort.

80. They vanish for days or weeks at a time and become unreachable, and you don't know where they are.

81. Your life is full of confusion and drama, and you don't understand why it never seems to be over.

82. You sound like you're losing yourself in a friendship.

83. You no longer know yourself.

84. Your life feels like it's at a standstill. You no longer have any hobbies or other passions. Your whole life revolves around them.

85. You sound like you're going nuts.

86. You may have considered suicide because you can't work out how to leave the relationship.

87. You mean, something is really wrong, and you knew something was wrong with them a long time ago, but you can't seem to get your mind around what or why they can't just stop behaving like that.

88. The relationship has changed, and you're not sure why or how, but details that were all right at the beginning of the relationship are not. It's like it's all twisted inside out.

89. Often, they're behaving like the person you know and pledge to improve, and you're curious if it would be different this time, but there's still a feeling of doubt that they're always up to the same things they've always been.

90. You don't take care of something and don't take care of anything—your life, your relationship, your partner, the world—and you just want to take care of stuff.

91. You're also advised that things you say and do are false.

92. You're arguing about the same thing over and over, and they just seem to be able to put themselves in your shoes and appreciate your viewpoint.

93. They do things you're not "allowed" to do.

94. They make you feel guilty about things that have never happened before or for having regular human responses to insane circumstances.

95. You find yourself playing an investigator, and you have such a deep gut instinct that the stuff they're telling you are lies, and you're beginning to figure out what they're doing.

96. You have thoughts that don't match the emotions you have; for example, you feel like you want to leave the relationship, but for some reason, you think you should stay close to them.

97. They treat you as if you're inferior to them, and you don't owe things like explanations or dignity.

98. They're rewording what you said and turning your words into meanings that you never meant, and no matter what you say, you can't persuade them that it's not what you meant or intended.

99. They make what you want to do too uncomfortable or impossible if you want to do it by doing a lot of things on this list, much of which could have gone unnoticed for a long time). Later, they insist they never stopped you from doing it, leaving you to feel uncertain over why you felt like they were stopping you.

100. You sound like you're going to lose your sanity.

Handling a Narcissist Boss

It can be very difficult to work with a manager who seems to be recovering from the NPD. Though you do not know for sure whether anyone else fits the requirements for a psychiatric diagnosis, you are likely to be well aware that they show the following types of characteristics:

- Insistency on being "right" all the way

- Can easily move from one extreme to treating you as the greatest worker on the planet, and the next moment may be trying to fire you in front of the board of directors, and back again on the basis of their present attitude and how they feel about you right now.

- Failure to cope with any conflict or assertion that there may be another way to do things, even though they brag about their "open door" policy.

- Lack of object constancy (for example, when they're upset with you, they may behave as though they can't recall any past good emotions about you and/or your job, and they may even try to fire you when they're angry with you).

- In need of continuous admiration, paired with excessive prevention and/or punishing actions when they do not feel adequately admired, otherwise shamed, embarrassed, or disrespected.

- They are frequently comparing employees who might also appear to be accidentally or deliberately pitting them against each other, often causing discord, animosity, and loss of solidarity within employees who are often focused solely on preserving their own careers.

- Can be highly aggressive, with people who work with them with people on their side, or even with their own supervisor.

Many people spend so many hours at work that their relationships with their supervisor, the way they feel about their performance, and their external opinions about it can be very critical to the overall emotional health and self-esteem.

Although all of this may be accurate, it's not really practical for people to leave their jobs, nor do they really want to, and asking the boss about it may lead to reprimand or firing. If your objective is to stay at your current job and do your best to coexist with your new employer, here's the bare bone version of mine.

Tips for Dealing With A Narcissist Boss:

Aim to make them look pretty good:

This could include moving above what they want (even though they ask in an irritating way), not giving them a bad mouth to superiors (even though they egg you on and being invaluable to them.

Research and Excel in what is Important to Them:

Your manager is likely to have special tasks that they like handled correctly ("or else") and other things that are very negative to them. Study what these items are and behave accordingly (even though it sounds stupid or unimportant to you).

Using Emotional Toolbox:

It can be very hard to be frequently insulted, no matter how hard you try, treated like trash, whether the manager is in a poor mood, or flipped to the drop of a hat. For this cause, it is really important to be extra kind to yourself and to do things that can make you feel stronger and preserve your self-esteem in this tough environment. This could include: constructive self-talk, taking brief breaks to breathe, and re-grouping, leaving early or remaining late when your supervisor leaves so that you can work better while it's quieter, preparing enjoyable activities for yourself before or after work, making time for exercising (even if it's a fast stroll around the block at lunch), etc.

Work to Stop Harming them Narcissistically

Bosses who suffer from NPD are particularly susceptible to narcissistic damage and are typically unable to cope calmly with something that feels: confrontational, humiliating, insubordinate, rude, or otherwise insulting. Of course, no one loves these emotions, but narcissists seem to respond especially violently and adversely, and it is doubtful that the object would be consistent in matching these kinds of negative feelings with some previously favorable ones about you, sometimes making them feeling negative about you and your work.

Keep Concentrated on the Objectives:

A lot of people may conclude that it's not worth getting their manager to deal with this everyday activity. On the other hand, this work may be an important move ahead in your future, or it may have other beneficial advantages that help you decide to continue. This is an independent decision for a person to make, regardless of what other people think is the right thing to do If you chose to stay, it would be immensely useful to make a list of all the stuff you're going to get out of leaving, how this work suits your needs in every way and the advantages you have of dealing with it. On days when it is especially difficult to work with your manager, please refer back to your list of reasons why you want to work there. This will act as a reminder that you're not only the villain here but that you can instead continue to concentrate your attention on the rewards of being there with you.

It can be incredibly difficult to function with a narcissist and to cope with the possible negative emotional consequences for you—the self-esteem, your level of fear, etc. The good news is that the more you learn about NPD and its general emotional and behavioral trends (as well as the particular patterns, interests, idiosyncrasies of this person), the more predictable your supervisor can get, and it's typically easier to deal with them. Assuming you plan to remain in your current position, note that this is your decision, you can set your limits, and most importantly, just because your boss calls you crazy, it doesn't necessarily mean you are.

Life with a Narcissist Partner

The narcissism will leave you feeling like you have met your true friend and soul mate. Everything's going to go fast. He's going to seem to fall in love quickly, and he's going to step in fast. At first, he might ask you to keep your relationship a secret because someone else in his life is over-controlling, doesn't approve of you, etc. And he doesn't want them to try to ruin this wonderful friendship that the two of you have with their envy or animosity.

Yet he's on the agenda. During this time, you should be confident that there is another woman in his life who is trapped with him in the evaluation process, and she has no idea about you. And she's not going to find out until she can work out how to make your relationship public, in the most dramatic, most hurtful way imaginable, during her discard. He's not going to be happy to break up with her, he's going to kill her, and you're going to be the tool he's going to use to do that. And deep down, that's just what he believes women deserve.

During the love-bombing, he'll tell you that you're different from any other woman in his world. He's going to complain about the other women, how needy they are, how mad they are, how usually feminine they are but not you. You're a special man. Well, you understand him. You're more than a human. He never thought, and will never see, any woman the way he feels for you.

And then, mysteriously, things appear to change. And with every step of the transition, your soul will be torn down a little further until you feel like a hollow, worthless shell as it sets you up for devaluation and discarding.

It's starting slowly. You start to be omitted first. And if you get angry, he tells you that it's not his fault; it's because the other people he's dealing with or friends with are jealous of you and don't understand. They're just trying to spare their emotions. If it were up to the narco, you'd be included, of course.

He's trying to motivate you to act the way he needs you to behave. He's going to thank you for the actions that would eventually make his plans simpler. He would admire your willingness to trust him enough to allow him independence, to sit at home, and to take care of the girls, so that he can go out and deal with his jobs. And it's still "work" regardless of whether it really is, how late it's going, how long it's going on, or how many days or continents it's going on. He's not on a break with his friends, and he's on a business trip. No matter what images your friends share on social media, you can be led to believe.

If you had any arguments with the narco, either he will flat out refute what he said or what he did, or he will accuse you of misinterpreting him since you're a typical woman and unable to understand what he really said. What you hear is what you think he meant. You're never listening to him. He's not unwise with you; you're unwise with him.

It's just about the projection, the gaslighting, the deflection of the narco. If he does to you, he's going to accuse you of doing to him. And he's going to tell everyone around you if he feels they're important enough.

If somebody is already talking about you until he's done (which they obviously won't be), you might learn that you're the one lying to him, that you're gasping him, that you're blaming him without evidence, that you're short-tempered with him that you're whining to friends about him that you're trying to turn people against him that you're trying to manipulate him, that you're trying to ruin his life and his livelihood, that's everything he's ever received. The list keeps moving on and on. This is a projection, and you should be confident that all the accuses you of doing to him is what he does to you, whether you know it or not.

And if you do or utter something that displeases the narco during your relationship together, it will make you regret it. He's going to get his pound of meat when he catches you and harangues you for hours on the smallest offense—for your own benefit, of course, to get you back in line. If you try to turn that into a two-way conversation, it'll piss him off even more, and the dressing-down can take another day or longer.

What he wants is for you to say he was right, you were wrong, and to feed him your guilt. And then note that he's always right, you're always wrong, and you're always mindful of your position. If you succeed in entering into some sort of discussion with the narco, you won't listen to the complexities of your argument or really know what you're really doing. He's going to skip straight to the worst situation, the most drastic circumstance possible, as a way to show, once and for all, that he's right and you're wrong.

Or he's going to respond to you with such a convoluted exercise in word salad that's too off the top and ridiculous and impossible to understand (or read), it's just better to agree with anything he says and not criticize him again ever, rather than having to go through all that again. And you can find that he begins to use amorphous 'others in his critique of you. Some people have observed your behavior. Some people have been complaining about you. Some people dislike you, and they're all your FAULT.

You're the source of all evil. You're bad. You're a bad guy, man. You're a hollow skeleton, and ALL OF That IS YOUR FAULT. And it's not just him that notices this in you. They're what he knows. Really, if it wasn't about him, you wouldn't have any friends at all. He's the one that goes on smoothing the route. He's the one who really needs to apologize to you and make excuses for you. He's the one that stops these amorphous others from even understanding how bad you are and disdaining you any more.

Around this time, he will also continue to be more discreet and then accuse you of not being available to him. He's not going to tell you what he's doing or where he's going, but he's going to ask you to tell him anything and then accuse you of never telling him. He's trying to suggest that if you don't tell him, he doesn't have to inform you about it. And if you wrote it all down on the family calendar, like he asked, well, how was he supposed to know? He's a young, important guy; he doesn't have time to review his calendars.

Then he starts securing the secret and makes sure that his computer, iPad, and phone are never left where you can reach it. Ok, congratulations. You're in the midst of the devaluation of hell.

And one day, when you walk into his party of friends, you're going to feel the glares and knives in your back. Some can also turn around and walk away from you. And you're starting to wonder what the heck you've ever done to them. Especially if you felt they were friends of yours too. They're not there.

The narco has been running to his groupies on a regular basis, telling them how abusive you are, how psychotic you are, how awful you are, how dishonest you are, how micro-managing you are, how you take advantage of him all the time, how you never listen to him how you need to be handled and monitored, or how you could ruin his life and his future.

He's going to take everything and anything you've ever said out of proportion and then exaggerate everything to the extent of becoming unrecognizable; the better he's going to flog you with it. After being rejoiced about how awful you are, how horrible you've always been, and given these distorted, exaggerated descriptions of what you're meant to be doing, they're going to endorse him one hundred percent. And then he'll use that encouragement to tell you he's clearly right about you because of look at how many people he's got on his side.

By the time it's over, the narco would have totally ruined your reputation and whatever emotions of friendship those mates might have felt for you. And they're his mates now and just his own. To the women, the narco is coming across as this vulnerable little boy who wants to be mothered and cherished and shielded from the huge, evil of you. To the guys, he's a comrade in arms who are being victimized by a slut, and they're going to have to band together.

And he'll have done all this for a surprisingly long time—after all these seeds have to be deliberately planted—and all behind your back. That way, he's able to get his next source of supplies on the hook-like your former friend who only wants this sad little lost boy to be his mum. When he's got her well and truly addicted, and he's in a relationship with her, he will plunge further into the devaluation and dump you, and do so in the cruelest way he sees fit.

And you stand there, totally flummoxed, wondering how your narco, who had just recently professed his undying affection, and how all your mutual friends could suddenly be so cold and overtly hostile to you. What have you ever done to any of them?

You could find one or two of them to say they're really your mates because they're going to ask you all kinds of personal questions, and you're going to answer them because you're so puzzled about what's going on because you want someone— anyone—to help you make sense of it. But for you, they're not there. They dig on behalf of the narco and see a) how well the devaluation is going and b) if there is something the narco wants to do to subvert you or to refute what you may say. Don't forget, and they're there to protect the narco. The narco is their world, just like it was yours, just a short time ago.

He's trying to turn anyone he can against you—friends, family members, even infants. For him, it's not about sanity or doing what's right for the girls, and it's about winning. It's just about killing you. It's about shaming you for being a woman and for wanting everything that you need. He resents you, he's upset at you, he hates you, and it's not because of what you've really done, but because of who you are and who you're not.

He's going to separate you from everyone you meet, or he's going to try. Whether he can drive you over the breaking point, it's just another evidence of how unfit you are. And he's never going to feel guilty for something he does to you, and it's all going to be your fault. He's trying to do the discard in the worst moment ever, or in the most drastic manner possible, and he needs to multiply the cut a thousand times, and that's what he thinks you deserve. Never mind if you stood by him, stood up for him, fulfilled all his desires, or lost everything for him. Now that the love-bombing is over, what he feels when he sees you is how pitiful you are and how deserving of his disdain.

That's when he actually takes out an irrevocable act to cause a discard, intended not just to end the relationship but to kill you. And that generally has to do with the way you think of your replacement. He might also scheme for you to trap them in the act if he knows he's going to have the most pain for you. But whatever he does, he's going to blame you for it. It's all going to be your fault, and thank god he had the presence of mind to triangulate in a new source.

This new woman—probably a close acquaintance of yours, or maybe a relative of yours—is so different from the other woman in her life. She's great, she's special, and no matter what stuff she does to you or your baby, she's the pinnacle of excellence. She's smarter than you are, she's better than you are, she's more in tune with him than you are, she's certainly up on the ladder of evolution than you are. And if you dare to utter her name with anything but respect and respect, he will come down upon you with all the wrath at his disposal. He wants you, in an odd way, to be pleased with his current source. If you dare to express any feeling, such as rage or confusion, he will double his devaluation towards you before he makes your life a living hell.

But before you find out about the new source, he's going to keep stringing you along, convincing you that if you just changed x, y, and z about your actions, the golden days of your relationship will come back. Why? Why? Since he loves watching you leap through hoops, and most importantly, your hoop-jumping keeps you out of his hair, so that he can go on with his plans. If you call him for some of his narco-behavior, particularly during the devaluation or discard periods, he will use the silent treatment or even take a few steps forward to go with the missed treatment.

It's a way to let him see how little you mean to him. He's trying to treat other people magnanimously in front of you—even people he usually can't stand—to hammer the point home on how even his rivals are worth more than you. You matter less than zero to him, and that's all your fault. Narcissists are beautiful, attractive people who make you feel like you've won some kind of love lottery. But dating a narcissist is a soul-sucking nightmare that's all about loneliness, breaking down your self-esteem, undermining your confidence, punishing you over and over for no apparent reason while trying to dangle a carrot of hope in front of you.

Why we Fall for a Narcissist

At one time or another, all of us will find ourselves dwelling on or healing from a romantic run-in with a narcissist. Suppose it was a brief or long-term engagement. In that case, it's possible that during the relationship post-mortem, you'll ask yourself how you managed to get pulled in by his or her charms, how you ignored all the warning signals, what made you so prone to the enchantments of a cold-hearted manipulator (and sometimes a cheat). It's generally not much consolation to know that these are actually the same questions that Echo's hapless nymph questioned herself after her meeting with the original Narcissus of Greek myth.

Why is it so easy to be Seduced by a Narcissist?

The short answer: nothing the narcissist does or does appears to be, and he or she is very, very good at manipulation—and, at least at the beginning of stuff, very charming and entertaining. The longer response is focused on the analysis of how narcissists work in partnerships. Five lessons science has learned from narcissists. The results are both revealing and cautious. Find the following:

The Same Attributes that Make Someone a Narcissist Account for his Initial Appeal

It's at this point where you should hopefully note that old lesson: don't judge a book by its cover. Narcissists exude self-confidence—a grandiosity fuelled by a heartfelt sense of entitlement—and they will do all they can to make you snow so that you become the admirer they crave. Researcher Mitja Back and collaborators have published experiments to find out why a narcissist makes such a perfect first impression. One of the factors is self-representation. Since narcissists are more about self-validating, they concentrate on appearance, including their clothing, grooming, and accessories. (My own narcissist drove a Porsche and wore very costly clothes.) Few of them are born physically beautiful, but they all struggle to retain a flawless and attractive appearance. Self-presentation also attracts favorable attention to them—whether in a dramatic or dominant style, wawing you with laughter, or captivating you with a shimmering chat, an easy smile, and beautiful manners—because a narcissist wants an audience to succeed.

And that's precisely what the studies revealed. In one sample of 72 freshmen—all meeting for the first time and therefore unfamiliar to each other—the researchers made each of them stand up and present themselves to the community after conducting the Narcissistic Personality Inventory. The others measured each individual in terms of looks, stylishness, attitude, and popularity. The latter was measured by questioning whether the person was likable and whether the observer wished to get to know the person.

Will it surprise you to hear that the narcissists were found the most beautiful and charming? All of us would feel ourselves squirming and nervous when we reveal ourselves to a room full of people, but not the narcissist, who, as the researchers called it, is "socially bold." A second experiment gave another audience a video of self-presentation from the first study, and again the narcissist scored a great deal of notoriety.

Boldness and the Feeling of Superiority Make the Narcissist Seem Attractive and Pretend to be a Good Friend

That's what Michael Dufner and others have discovered in a series of studies. In reality, they sent male participants into the streets of a German city with the challenge of contacting 25 women—random strangers—and getting their phone numbers, email addresses, and other contact details. Study assistants accompanied the men and then interviewed the people they had met, asking if they enjoyed the interaction and the conversation, if they liked the man, and if they were drawn to him. True enough, the more arrogant the guy was the more contacts he made, and the more desirable he appeared to women.

The narcissist clearly knows how to make things happen. Alas, while the show seems to be aimed at the person he or she is with, it's not just about them. It's just about self-affirmation. But it takes longer for the narcissist's wife to find it out.

The Narcissist is a Game-Playing Specialist

Studies suggest that narcissists like partners but choose short-term relationships without commitment. They appear to look for the next bond that matches their desires when they're already in a relationship, so it's quite likely that they're cheating on their current love interest. One of the reasons why narcissists will cause their wives a lot of emotional harm is all the mixed signals: the narcissist needs to be in a relationship—but just on his own terms.

Their type of partnership, including the work of W. Keith Campbell and others, has proven that it is the game-play that gives them the leverage of the partnership and their mate. They enjoy control and defend their autonomy—avoiding true affection and commitment—but they do want your attention and sexual gratification. It's like living in a mirror house, except that the only mirror that matters is the one the narcissist keeps in his palm.

At the conclusion of their article, Campbell and his collaborators were asked whether anybody would be dating a narcissist. They must observe that with the beauty and charisma of the narcissist, it needs the patience to be wise in his or her strategies. They also venture that narcissists can target people who are low in self-esteem—on the surface, narcissists look like major captures, after all—and who are vulnerable to self-doubt. Alas, it's a plain fact that when a genuine person gets mixed up with someone who plays sports, it's a sincere person that's going to get hurt.

At a Technical Level, the Narcissist can be really Nice in Bed

James K. McNulty and Laura Widman's work primarily looks at how narcissism works in the sexual domain—because, as they write, "Having a high-quality sexual relationship is an integral part of having a high-quality romantic relationship." What's fascinating is that, sexually, narcissists are a rather mixed bag. They lack sympathy for their partners, but evidence suggests that empathy is part of a healthy sexual experience. Open contact is part of healthy sex, but the self-focused narcissist is not involved in open communication. They also note that narcissists appear to be sexually abusive and prefer infidelity—a behavior that is adverse to a healthy romantic relationship.

But here comes the seductive force of the narcissist, together with the mental uncertainty he or she will shower about your life: narcissists enjoy women, and they're really concentrated on how successful they are about anything. So being "good in bed" matters a lot to them. In the sexual realm, the narcissistic characteristics that are triggered are an entitlement, exploitation, and an increased sense of skill. McNulty and Widman's marriage happiness research have reinforced all of these conclusions regarding narcissists—both negatives about contact and affection and positive results about sexual abilities.

However, a second analysis by these authors indicated that it was sexual narcissism, not generalized narcissism, that projected infidelity. It is estimated that 25 percent of married men and 20 percent of married women cheat—so clearly, not all cheaters are narcissists. McNulty and Widman found that a sense of sexual superiority, confidence in sexual capacity, and lack of sexual sympathy towards a partner were related to infidelity.

The Narcissist does not Apologize or Forget

There is another reason why the relationship with the narcissist is going to be rocky: according to the work of Julie Juola Exline and others, dispute resolution is almost difficult with the narcissists since they are cynical about the importance of forgiveness on the one side and easily insulted on the other. They prefer to do a cost-benefit analysis where there has been a transgression of some kind in a relationship and usually do not see the benefit of either forgiving or ignoring. They're quick to hang on to a grudge.

How a Narcissist Target and Control You

Narcissists have become self-absorbed. They also control interactions, exploit their loved ones, and engage in manipulative profit-making behavior. We strive to get rid of these fake people, but we still fall prey to their abuse. So how are they going to do this? How do narcissists dominate you? What kind of techniques do they use? Here are five strategies used by narcissists to monitor their targets:

1. They're Hitting Codependents

Narcissists also have success in manipulating people when they are exploiting codependents. "Overall, narcissists seek out those with characteristics of codependence," states Tom Gagliano, Relationship Specialist. "The narcissist emphasizes the vulnerabilities of the codependent, that they are conditioned to feel that it is their fault or that they are responsible for correcting any dissatisfaction throughout the partnership. The companion is terrified of the narcissist to the point that they lose their sense of themselves by trusting in all the distortions of the narcissist."

2. They Make you Feel Unique about it

These self-centered people often go out of their way to make others feel special—not because they actually admire something about the person, but because they exploit it. "In their relationships, narcissists often gain control of others by playing with a person's (very understandable) desire to feel special and highly valued," says Clinical Psychologist Forrest Talley. "The narcissist might say, for example, 'Though I just met you, it is obvious to me that you are incredibly bright and competent. I have a very small group of people, much like you, who I want to stay in touch with... I want you to be part of that group. Only give me your phone number, and I'll add it to my special black book.' (Sound ridiculous? That's it because that's what a narcissist told me years ago... no, not a patient)."

3. They're Using Shock, Anxiety, and Guilt

Narcissists continue to take control over people in their lives by evoking difficult feelings. "After a period of 'grooming' someone for a close relationship, the narcissist moves on to use shock, fear, and guilt to maintain control," Talley explains. "The outrage and awe come from the over-the-top, emotionally fraught tantrums that erupt when a mate (spouse or lover) does something that disappoints the narcissist. Most rational people find such dramatic responses stressful and unusual, so they begin to work hard to prevent a repeat show."

4. They're Gaslight

Narcissists are often commonly gas lighters, which means they are expert manipulators. "Gaslighting is the tactics of narcissists, sociopaths, and psychologists," says Christine Scott-Hudson, Certified Psychotherapist. It is a narcissistic activity built for self-giving and also for sport. It's built to weaken, deceive, and destabilize the victim. Gaslighters can argue that they said anything or did something you know they said or did. They're going around the universe unhappily."

5. They're Playing Hot and Cold Football

In the end, selfish people are also apt to play sports. "One of the ways narcissists try to control you is by playing manipulative hot and cold games," says Adina Mahalli, Master Social Worker. "One week, they're going to flatter you to get you to do what they want; the next week, they're going to use violence. The bad moments are interspersed with positive moments so that you do not even know that you are being fooled. The only way to defeat this is to be vigilant when it comes to flattery and positivity. They take a move with a grain of salt and don't let love-bombing be a kind of extortion to you. Niceties aren't meant to be conditional."

Be conscious of these five common techniques of narcissists. If you suspect you've been killed or threatened by these manipulators, do what you can to get them out of their reach. This could mean breaking ties with friends or family members— but that's all right because your mental wellbeing and well-being are on the line, and that's always a priority.

Don't be an Easy Victim for a Narcissist

If you've found yourself a survivor of narcissistic violence, here's the truth: none of it was your fault, and narcissists are the greatest emotional abusers. Chances are you've heard about Narcissistic Personality Disorder so far, but someone doesn't have to have a full-blown NPD case to have the narcissistic characteristics to make them risky to get interested.

It could almost appear like you weren't involved with him, rather that he was involved with you. One day you flirted with this man who you thought was amazing, and the next thing you knew, you were in an immediately serious and dedicated relationship, and you can't remember exactly how that happened.

This is because narcissists are the masters of survival. It's because they have the sixth sense to recognize people with personality characteristics that make them more likely to fall to the charismatic person of the narcissist and to hang around to take care of them long though they show their repulsive inner self. This is where learning how to deal with a narcissist will motivate you to get them out of your life.

But do you know the symptoms of narcissistic personality disorder? If you can associate with the attributes of the 7 points below, you might be at a greater than normal risk of being pursued by a narcissist.

1. You Have Something the Narcissist Wants (Money, Power, Position, Lifestyle)

There is a special dynamic that comes into play in a partnership where a narcissist is engaged. It begins with a hook— a fantasy, sometimes one you believe is for you, but it's just about power for the narcissist.

Often the narcissist will come off as supportive, and then when things don't work out, the table will turn on you. If you've caught up or managed to get him to take action, the stress just escalates.

2. You have a Caregiver's Nature and a Strong Need to Help Others

The partnership appears to be a match made in heaven for a moment, but it's a short ticket to hell. The generosity and goodness of the caretaker are reflected in the early stages of the relationship. The giver has others to do so because being the core of the world fits perfectly for the selfish desires of an emotional vampire. Yet as the relationship grows more personal, the narcissist consumes the time, attention, and money of the relationship while maintaining power.

3. You have a Compassionate, Empathetic Disposition

Narcissists have a justification behind all that happens in their lives, and it is really their own fault. Of course, you listen, and you want to help, but if you hear yourself thinking, "I was just trying to be nice..." more and more frequently, and if any of you get used to it, odds are there's a bad dynamic at hand. In reality, empathic personalities and caretaker forms are ideal candidates for emotional vampires.

4. You Grew up in a Dysfunctional Environment

Your past can make it hard to spot border violations when they happen, which may lead you to disregard your gut instincts whenever anyone breaks your trust. Narcissists don't like borders. Suppose a person has an inability to set them, hold them, or take responsibility after one has been abused. In that case, the predatory form detects the vulnerability and uses it to their benefit. Often narcissists commit valiant deeds; however, instead of promoting their partner's individuality or empowerment, they utilize their support as a method of establishing dependency.

5. You are Lonely and Feel a Desperate Need to Find Love

Find a desire, satisfy a need" is the slogan of the narcissist. An individual with poor self-esteem is simpler to manage than anyone with a strong sense of self-confidence. At first, the force sounds nice, so it may be mistaken with love, yet the narcissist is incapable of honesty. Slowly the passion wanes, and the cold, calculating demeanor leaves you asking what went wrong and seeking to find the caring person you thought you met.

6. You Willingly Accept Blame — even for Things You didn't Do

If the relationship deteriorates, narcissists use shame to "prove" that you are the issue. Empathetic and emotional people are highly vulnerable to gambling as a function of their reflective nature. By redirecting your focus to something you have "wrong," done, the narcissist distracts people away from their own unhealthful conduct.

7. Avoid Conflict and Confrontation

Narcissists prey on paranoia and use it to build smoke screens and mirrors. Non-confrontational individuals are always fearful of abandonment, shame, or something that could contribute to the end of an important friendship. When narcissists respond aggressively, these fears are triggered by those who are bent backward to keep things orderly and peaceful. Counter-intuitively, the more confrontation you stop, the more appealing you become to a narcissist.

You wouldn't have to be a survivor yet. Draw from what you've learned from your past and empower your instincts so that in the future, you'll know how to stop another narcissist if you're targeted. Listen to your intuition, trust your heart, and know that if it's too good to be true, it's a chance.

PART 3: RECOVERING FROM NARCISSIST ABUSE

How do I Heal from Cognitive Dissonance after a Narcissistic Relationship?

Cognitive Dissonance (CD) is the frustration that happens when we don't grasp the acts or conduct of our own or anyone else. We don't understand that anything about these behavior violates our beliefs about ourselves, about them, or about people and the universe. We may minimize discomfort in three ways: change our actions, our values, and/or our memories.

Ns is a specialist in reducing the shipload of CDs that would arise if they could see themselves without protective blinkers. They usually do this by allowing reflexive use of exaggeration, projection, and denial-an an extraordinary and breathtaking capacity to forget details and re-shape memory and truth to meet their needs. And just by lies. Are they really' forgetting, or are they really trying to? It's new. It doesn't matter to you. It's the same thing about you.

For instance, you've just made a novel, out-of-the-box idea to your manager about how to cope with a complicated problem that affects everyone on the team. You have presented a very unique and innovative solution to the issue, but with a very good chance of succeeding. Your manager considers this for a second, and looks to you straight-faced and says, "I think we should do this." She continues to propose the Same plan of action you've just proposed. However, she proposes this-to you, right after you've suggested it! -as fresh ideas and reflections of her own. She also advises that you take the notes! If you say, "You know, do you think we should do what I just suggested? "(As you would have done the first few times), she's going to look at you blankly.

She's acknowledged the importance of your advice, can't handle the CD by knowing that you've come up with a brilliant concept that's going to save the day all. The positive ideas come from her! -and now she just instantly-somehow-makes these thoughts her own. You're gob-smacked the first time this happens and frankly don't know what to do about it, but after a few occasions and bringing stuff together about other odd facets of her actions, you're beginning to understand.

Non-Ns strive to minimize the CD they experience in this kind of situation by different kinds of mental gymnastics-rationalizations, etc. When we exhaust all the other options and confess to ourselves that (incredible as it seems) someone is actually re-writing history as they go (always in a manner that flatters themselves and absolves them of any blame or deficiency), we begin to realize that the person we're working with has some very odd things going on and cannot be trusted.

We begin to understand how they can depend so strongly on us and need us so desperately, still not be able to respect us-not only us or others but ourselves. In reality, the more positive ideas we have and the stronger our job, the more they feel the need to devalue, verbally harass, and undermine us. Colleagues who have found that they begin to make subtle comments out of respect for us are commendable. At that point, we should either avoid being helpful (at this point, they may be nicer to us), affirm their distortions (tell them how smart they are and how much you've gained from them-that is, drink the kool-aid, or make them think we have), endure their disrespect and utter lack of concern for us or end the partnership. We should try to encourage them to understand themselves, too. I tried this incredibly difficult and risky, and I made them hate me more.

Unfortunately, the operation of defense mechanisms is usually not that simple or easy to detect. It could take a long time if this kind of stuff is new to us. We spend all sorts of time wondering why they don't appear to appreciate our job, wondering, challenging ourselves and our assumptions, and even starting to doubt our own comprehension and memory and vision.

This is bad enough in a professional relationship, and once you realize the intense defense processes at work in narcissism, you will miss a lot of sleep. When you're in a romantic relationship with someone, it's a lot tougher. We've got a lot at stake, and our mental gymnastics are getting serious.

We can't help seeking brief comfort by drinking the N kool-aid-sometimes over and over. They are nice and sweet, no matter how unethical their acts are-because they are sometimes, and when it's good, it's so good and comforting to us. We seek comfort in the same friendship that is causing us agony. But then the CD returns, even at 'normal hours, causing considerable emotional and, in many instances, serious physical distress-after we have been seriously injured many times. Things may be going fine, but it's our unconscious prods to remember to keep on watch. Dreams and nightmares tend to say it as it is, that physical discomfort and unease continue to arise in their presence, or even when we think about them. We may have nausea and fear. Listen to your body, man!

We may be going the way of trying to justify it to ourselves-but. This is both complicated and risky. And ultimately, we see that their needs-their essential lies-will still override our interest when their egos or reputations or pride are challenged. Or if they want anything and care for us is in the way, and our options are made clear at that point.

We put up with it, dwindling ourselves poorly and putting ourselves at great risk-because they're going to chuck us under the bus when it suits them. We're going to stay in the situation and drink the kool-aid-either obviously or honestly. Or we're going to get out.

How are we healing? By knowing what's going on with them. And then realizing that they are what they are, that we're not at fault, recognizing that saving them comes at too high a cost, and accepting that in any case, we're over our heads. Over everything by running out of here. And then by not worrying about it, particularly if we have difficulty believing that certain people have little to no guilt or compassion. It's a very tough thing for some people to consider. That was because of me. It's already there.

The Healing Process

Narcissist Personality Disordered men and women are so difficult to connect to since they are incapable of truly knowing you and incapable of caring about you and your emotions. The same is true of their offspring. But I've been bringing together the stuff that has helped me cope with the NPD/ASPD Mask for 47 years. Remember that they are emotionally ill and unable to adjust where they can have a mature, positive, caring, and loving relationship.

Here are some of the items that I find to be useful in knowing and maintaining coping mechanisms following the Narcissist's final discard or quitting them. You're continuing the trip on the road to recovery.

It's not your fault! In this marriage, you did nothing wrong to deserve this mental, verbal, sexual, or physical violence. You can move ahead to marry someone else and enjoy a satisfying relationship, but they will never be able to do so effectively.

You're not alone in this. I know that you feel alone and alone because your support systems have never lived behind closed doors of the NPD then they don't appreciate your spouse's incredibly nuanced and dishonest actions or something else you've had to experience. That's why I'm here to help you get through quitting the NPD and healing.

Educate Yourself on NPD

Discover all the characteristics and deceptive habits of the NPD, so you can avoid them and any potential NPD you encounter from becoming a survivor. This was the most important step to complete for me. You're a kind and compassionate guy; otherwise, he wouldn't have targeted you because he doesn't have those characteristics. To get you into their fold, they "Love-Bombed" you into believing that you had the same beliefs, interests, and dislikes ambitions, and desires. They tell you, in truth, that you are "soulmates! "They tell you that all of you are so close and in love, so why wait, and you'll soon move in or get married. You need to educate yourself about what they're doing, how they're doing that, and why they're doing it. Now there are so many books, posts on the internet, and Quora is a wonderful source of learning their warped attitudes and thought. They're so different from the normal" behavior of a human being.

Self-Assessment

Evaluate If you were able to get sucked in their twisted & tangled web of deception and disinformation! It's not your fault that they are emotionally ill and deemed to be toxic. Yet, it will make you realize how you've been tricked into their culture. I had a wonderful friendship with my dad, so it was hard for me to accept my husband's relentless frustration with me. His love-bombing was because my parents were in love in real life, so it felt like they were on the surface. Yet behind closed doors, there was nothing but False LOVE and pure lies! You must realize why they have scammed you.

If you have children, then write down all incidences for each child that you can recall so that you can hopefully demonstrate how inept they are as a parent. They don't love your kids, nor do they care for their children. So I'd recommend you get full custody of your kid with no custody. Our courts are not up-to-date on these behavioral personality issues. This way, when diagnosing you, you have a witness and proof of how you have been handled, which can give the courts the edge of bending on your side, including all phone numbers, emails, other people who heard things, notes, email, and pictures explaining their actions. He's going to lie to the judge in court and think nothing about it. You've got to be prepared.

Seek out a doctor, preferably a doctor who has improved understanding of NPD behavior. It took me three years of weekly counseling to understand and recover from extreme depression, Complicated PTSD, significant chronic stress-related disorders, and Trauma Bonding (Stockholm Syndrome) induced by 47 years of NPD life.

Find an experienced attorney who knows NPD while you're going through a divorce. Also, strive to get the child's full custody because the NPD is not a responsible mom. They don't care or love the boy. They just want the kid to get back to you so they can make your life miserable. It's hard, but you've got to be entirely non-reactive for their actions. If they're going to get a response out of you, they enjoy it. But don't respond to something they do, even though you're horrified at what they say and do. Often don't confront them about their NPD characteristics; they don't care for you or how you feel. You need to understand that he's got 100 percent of you.

If you plan to leave, you don't need to go to No Contact when you dropped off the face of the earth. This means that under no conditions are you talking to them, calling them, writing them, or delivering any texts to them. Make them speak to your counsel about this. They're trying to do something to try to get you out. Avoid "all contact." means you're going to break off all contacts with them and move on in your life. The NPD is extremely aggressive and is known to be a master at exploiting and getting you back, which is why I suggest No Interaction because it is the most viable way to escape the NPD.

Why is no Contact Advised?

Once they are in touch with you, they will force you to come back, and their penalty will be harder when you come back. Since you left them once before, they're more determined; you won't abandon them a second time! It is also advised that you update all the passwords to your phone and to your computer. Changing the door locks, get new credit cards, a new mobile phone number, don't write, or even speak to them. Don't leave a hint of where you went to launch your new life.

You Deserve Joy and Pleasure

Don't close the door to a new guy in your life who will cherish the way a woman or a man should be loved. However, you need to find the time to get into a new relationship, and you need to recover. If you enter into a new relationship before you recover, you are likely to enter into another relationship with a narcissist. When you go through these steps, and complete your treatment, try to take the time to get back to yourself. It normally takes 18–36 months to recover. Don't panic if it takes longer. You're going to recover a bit older, but a lot smarter. You're going to get the confidence back. Allow them time to recover. Eventually, you need to unlock your soul's door. You're not going to shut it down forever.

What Made Me Safe?

What makes me strong are the two responses that teach me and trust God.

Educate Yourself on NPD

First of all, I've been arming myself with the awareness of NPD symptoms so that I can identify the signs clearly and learn how to run the other way should you see someone like this in the future. I read everything I could about the subject. It made me understand that once they get a full NPD blown, they're unlikely to get better.

Great Faith in Religion

The second quality I have discovered is my strong faith in believing God. God has given me the courage to survive what I've been through. As a result, I am now equipped with a lot of information on the recognition of characteristics related to Covered Narcissistic Personality Antisocial Personality Disorder. I grew up imagining my future as a college professor, but my life has changed drastically, and I'm learning to look at the bright side of my life. God has given me the opportunity to write and share my thoughts with others who are suffering, and I will support them to find their way to healing. If I can help improve my life, that's the 47 years I've wasted!

On Your Recovery Path!

Good luck to you on the way back to the journey of healing. Don't think if the time is shorter or longer. You can develop PTSD Complex, which is a post-traumatic stress disorder. Very definitely, if you are in a long-term relationship with the NPD, you are trauma bonded (Stockholm Syndrome). Don't let that intimidate you. It can be difficult, but it's important to understand and communicate with a trained therapist who understands personality problems, Nuanced PTSD, and Trauma Bonding.

They never loved you or cared about your feelings. They're incapable of ever loving you, and they could care less for your feelings. They're incapable of ever respecting you or even their children. They don't think for any of your emotions if you're lonely, upset, confused, angry, and they lack human sympathy. They're not successful parents, so try to get custody of the children. The only reason they want children to be in the care of you!

CONGRATULATIONS!

The NPD left you in the first step of quitting or becoming blessed. You are no doubt the target of the NPD, but the lone NPD SURVIVOR!! Best of luck to you, and you're strong. You deserve to be cherished and loved again! I'm going to pray for you if you get in touch with me

THE RACIAL HEALING

A guide for social justice. Overcome systemic racism, stop violence against unprotected categories and manage inequality issues within communities.

MARTIN JORDAN

"Prejudice is an opinion without judgment."

— Voltaire

"I plan to stand by nonviolence, because I have found it to be a philosophy of life that regulates not only my dealings in the struggle for racial justice, but also my dealings with people, and with my own self."

— Martin Luther King Jr.

INTRODUCTION

This manual dispenses the valid suggestions to undertake a step-by-step path to stem and overcome racism. Obviously, a historical social excursus on American society makes the book a complete work on a current and very involving topic. There is no shortage of anecdotes and curiosities that allow a compelling reading.

"The Racial Healing" wants to raise awareness of the history of racism and to protect the victims of prejudice, with the aim of providing the correct approach to stem and defeat racism. The more you know about the problem, the better you can deal with it.

Talking about this issue with people can cause some discomfort, because they face difficult truths. It must be remembered that the views of people who suffer from the negative effects of racism are legitimate and must be treated as such. Therefore it is fair to say forcefully that there are no races as far as people are concerned. These certainties must be widespread throughout the world, supported and defended at any price. Each of us must make it our own without having to feel guilty and without being defensive in expressing our own conviction.

The racist is one who suffers from an inferiority or superiority complex. The result is the same, because his behavior, in one case or another, will be of contempt. And from contempt, we go to anger. The common man reasons with his prejudices, in that he judges others even before knowing them. To combat fear, man sometimes provokes his aggression. He feels threatened and attacks. The racist is also the one who hates the foreigner because he feels disgusted. In any case, racism is a form of discrimination, something unjust or unreasonable. One does not have the right to believe that because of being white skin one has more quality than a black person.

Racism is dangerous because it does not give value to others' lifes and develops thanks to the preconceived ideas about peoples, from which the culture of fear arises, which very often flows into violence.

Fighting racism is a sociological and civil commitment, because the racist is at the same time a danger for others and a victim for himself. Racism is a fairly widespread behavior common to all men but it is not normal, natural behavior. It is an artificial construction of society, based on negative feelings, which inspire mistrust and then contempt for one's own kind, which have physical and cultural characteristics different from the dominant group.

A child becomes an adult racist based on the context in which he lives and the education received. In fact, if a child is educated by racist people he will become racist and it will be normal for him to be. Therefore, the fight against racism must be a daily reflection. We must not underestimate or neglect the little things, we must not let go, because these behaviors can develop and prosper even among people who could easily have avoided abandoning themselves to that scourge.

Racism claims that it doesn't matter to know a person's strengths and weaknesses, it is enough to know that he or she is part of a certain community to reject it. We must not overlook the fact that man's respect for his fellow man is essential for a harmonious civil coexistence and we must act as long as we are in time. Different people must not be discriminated against, because a multiracial society is an enrichment and an opportunity for everyone. Every life deserves respect, because everyone has the right to his dignity.

AMERICAN SOCIETY

According to the dominant narrative, the United States of America are based on a pluralistic society, tolerant of dissent and, above all, multicultural. The States is a nation founded on the union of former colonies dependent on several European nations. To this initial specificity the cultural identities of the various immigrants have been added, which have given shape to a complex social mix. Obviously it was a more conflict-prone society than an ethnically homogeneous society.

Before the civil war, the so-called assimilation effect was adopted for immigrants, with the obligation to learn the English language. With reference to this period, we speak of the Americanization of immigrants, who renounced the effects of multiculturalism, in favor of assimilating the dominant cultural forms.

Between the end of the nineteenth and the beginning of the twentieth century, in an attempt to manage the substantial migratory waves that hit the States, the optimistic image of the melting pot spread, characterized by groups of minority identities and with equal rights and a proactive vision of life. It was a particular model of multiethnic society, in which with the succession of generations, immigrants would be destined to merge with the population of the host country.

The word melting represents the process of fusion of different cultures which come together in the pot which represents the dominant culture. In American society, the pot is made up of the western European-derived corporate model, the so-called Wasp community, White-AngloSaxon-Protestant.

However, this project encounters strong resistance.

For decades the social life of immigrants was limited to contact with members of the same community, from work to marriage. Likewise, the presence of neighborhoods defined on an ethnic basis in most of the American metropolises "Little Italy", "Chinatown", testify to the failure of the integration operation.

There is no doubt, in fact, that the social movements of the sixties are also due to the failure of the policies led by the myth of the melting pot. The saddest consequence of this policy is represented by racial segregation which has generated and still generates bloody social conflicts.

It is no coincidence that during the 1960s a new image spread to describe the pluralism of American society, that of the salad bowl. It is a metaphor that refers to the ingredients of a salad which, even if mixed, maintains its initial characteristics.

The idea focuses on the coexistence of individuals and social groups who, with their own separate identities, manage to find the balance for proper integration with the indigenous population.

This process resulted in the formal recognition of identities such as American Europeans, African Americans, Asian Americans and Latin Americans. Since then there has been the spread of some regulatory tools the "affirmative actions", to promote social equality and to promote principles of racial, ethnic and sexual equity.

This initiative represents the turning point towards a real multiculturalism. On March 6, 1961, President Kennedy passed an executive order that the hiring would no longer be dictated by the color of the skin. Measures to facilitate access to universities for African American students followed. Recently, in favor of the rhetorical provision of the color-blind, a noble attempt to favor social mobility, these benefits have been suppressed naturally.

On the contrary, these policies have often produced harmful effects. There has been an increase in hostility and episodes of racism towards the African American community. The fact that African Americans and Latinos make up about 30% of the population, but they represent 60% of the prison population, is very significant, on the discrimination in the USA. Civil rights organizations report ethnic health disparities. African Americans die six times more than whites, as they receive less care, while doing jobs considered essential but low-income.

Politicians, civic rights activists and doctors have long argued that information on ethnicity is needed to ensure that all communities have equal access to testing and treatment and also to help develop a public health strategy to protect those who are more vulnerable.

Despite the myth of the melting pot and salad bowl, racism and discrimination are still rooted in American society. This testifies how sensitive American society is to the issue of diversity but, at the same time, poses the problem of racial disparities which emerges as an unresolved issue.

American society still seems far from reaching the Americanized racial identity desired by integration projects. The demographics do not reflect the myth of a color blind society and citizens continue to use specific ethnic categories to define themselves.

According to the latest census, Americans are ethnically much more diverse than in the past, mainly due to a further increase in immigration. In particular, Asia and Latin America are progressively establishing themselves, together with Africa, from which most of the immigrants come.

Ethnic-cultural diversity does not mean peaceful coexistence in any case. According to some studies, the color line that divides American society between blacks and whites, and that has characterized American society since its origins, seems to have even grown in recent years. Likewise, hate crimes against blacks, Latinos and immigrants from the Middle East are even on the rise compared to the past.

It is too simplistic to download everything about the Trump effect, as well as historically reductive. Although for a long time praised and observed only as a source of growth and wealth, the multiculturalism of American society is a decidedly problematic issue and inversely proportional to the stability of the country.

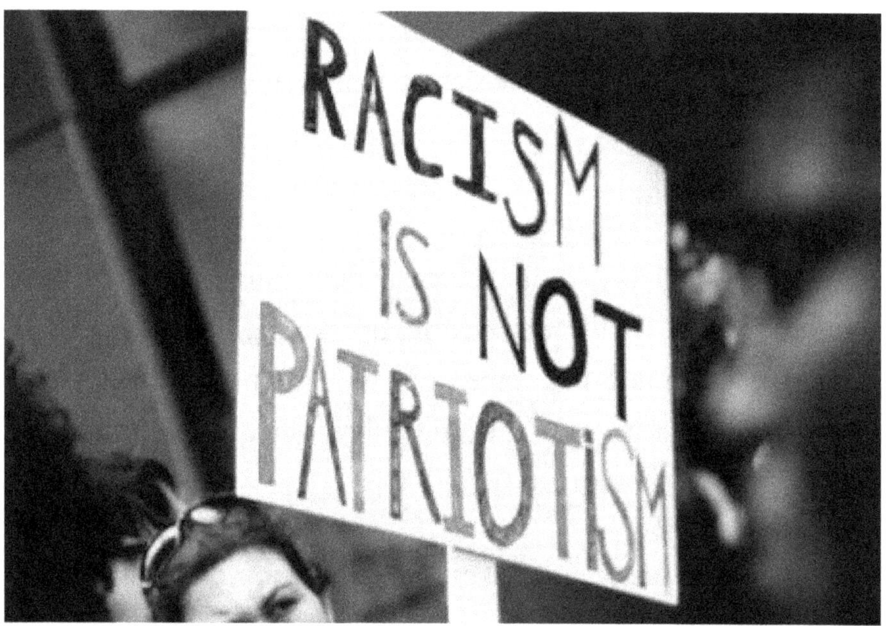

The lack of efficient policies could be instrumental in perpetrating their deep divisions. Each relationship with difference is characterized by variability, complexity and ambivalence. Without an ethical commitment on the part of the institutions to encourage dialogue between the parties, any political solution will prove counterproductive to the creation of national cohesion.

1. WHAT IS RACISM?

There are no human races.

The vision of humanity divided into upper and lower races in relation to a biological inheritance would derive from the predominance of some groups of people over others. For this reason, there were enormous social and political consequences for the development of human history.

Between the nineteenth and twentieth centuries, a broad debate began on the issue of race. However, the experts agreed that the real problem is not racial differences but rather the negative meaning attributed to racism, understood as the doctrine and practice of discrimination.

Biological theories of race underwent profound changes in the 1930s when, with the emergence of genetics, it could be said that there were potentially as many breeds as there were genes. It was documented that not the species but the gene was the selection unit and that the groups usually considered breeds were not biological phenomena but political inventions.

It would have been more correct to speak of ethnic groups instead of racial groups.

The most recent research in the field of genetics has demonstrated irrefutably that there are no different human races, but only one human species. Yet racism as a social phenomenon exists and has heavy repercussions for both the people concerned and social cohesion.

Discrimination against minority groups has a long tradition. Until the 17th century, these discriminatory practices drew justification above all from religious doctrines. During the eighteenth and nineteenth centuries theories divided human beings according to ethnicity, and into groups with hereditary characteristics, ultimately into biological races.

These theories gave birth to racist ideology, which is based on a reductive vision of human beings, classified on the basis of real or imaginary characteristics of a physiognomic or cultural type according to categories such as skin color, nationality and religion. Moreover, others are considered to be morally, culturally, intellectually or physically inferior beings.

Racism manifests itself in subtle forms of discrimination in everyday life and more structurally in the form of prejudices. The demeaning of a person targeted by a racist act corresponds to the strengthening of the dominant position of those who commit it, while in the victims it provokes aggressive or renunciationary reactions of social retreat.

Although the topic has been the subject of numerous studies, there is still no definition of the concept of racism unanimously recognized and shared. Classical racism starts from the construction and accentuation of real or imaginary differences between its victim and its executioner, which legitimizes an attack or a privilege to its advantage.

There is another definition, in a broader sense, based on cultural, psychological, social and metaphysical topics. People are not judged and treated as individuals, but as belonging to pseudo-natural groups, with collective characteristics deemed immutable. The breed social construct is not only based on external characteristics, but also on presumed cultural, religious and hereditary peculiarities.

An Artificial Construction

The object of racism is a creation of the modern world. Modern racism, in fact, was born for a transformation of pre-existing behaviors, in the continuous search for security mechanisms, through a political power that is based on discipline and control.

Racism, therefore, has to do with a modern power, which not only limits itself to regulating society but takes charge of the life and death of its citizens.

It is no coincidence that the modern world, with the excuse of regulating society, has witnessed the unleashing of the most complete murderous power.

The last century saw the genocide of Native Americans, Armenians, European Jews and gypsies, communists, homosexuals, physically and mentally disabled, pacifists, religious dissidents of various faiths.

Racism was the appropriate response to the practice of modern states to interfere with the lives and deaths of their citizens.

Foucault asserted that racism ensures the function of death and at the same time strengthens the biological and economic power of those who practice this perverse mechanism, as members of a race or population that believe themselves superior.

Racism is not a natural practice, it is the result of an artificial construction, which calls into question ourselves. If we want to refer to a metaphor, racism is like a mirror in which what we believe to be the face of our identity is reflected.

Sartre said in the pamphlet on anti-Semitism that the Jew is a human being whom others call Jewish. That pamphlet ended up in the hands of his teacher by Franz Fanon, who suggested that he replace the Hebrew word with the word neger. Like the Jew, even the black people, the colonized, the migrant, is the subject of an artificial creation that rejects it as anomalous and builds it as a carrier of natural characters.

The first step in this construction is the negation of its history. The difference appears suddenly without a history, a life, a pre-existing subjectivity. This void will be filled with pretext narratives, of which the degree of verisimilitude does not matter. Each racist assertion is based on one or more logical fallacies, on incorrect reasoning, deformed information.

Behind every racist assertion there is only a mind incapable of consequentiality, a subject who needs to believe in the absurdities he utters. These sad passions constitute the social practices that generate the racial problem.

The Jew was built from the medieval behaviors of the Christian Church. The concept of Jew bore the message that the alternative to the existing order brought chaos and devastation within itself. A world made up of nation states abhorred the void without national characters supported by the Jews.

The same reasoning applies to African-Americans, Asians and North American natives in the mid-nineteenth century. All the different, alien components of modern society had to be rationally constructed and narrated, controlled and managed.

Zygmunt Bauman claims that the modern, immune medical paradigm prevails. It is not important to establish the balance between pro-life and contrary functions. Here we see a paradigm at work in which we conceive the absurd idea of erasing the existence of an element different from the pre-established society.

Besides medicine, gardening also contributes to the mental form of modernity. Both disciplines, according to Bauman, participate in the construction of an artificial social order through the elimination of those elements of reality that do not fit into the perfect reality imagined by the dominant people.

As in gardening and medicine, it is a question of isolating the useful elements, destined to live and thrive, from the harmful and pathological ones, which like weeds and cancerous tissues must be suppressed.

The Heterophobia

Heterophobia, the emotional, passionate, instinctive fear of the other has to do with an object, the foreigner. He threatens the unity and identity of the indigenous group and erases all differences. However, genocides have occurred not only because of their aversion to diversity. Peculiar structures of modernity were needed to perpetrate the brutalities of the twentieth century, such as rationalism, principles of efficiency, planning of bureaucracy.

This means that we must be aware of the fact that the possibility of the Holocaust, as an exercise of the power of death on a large scale of populations, always remains latent.

The racist will be the one who does not question those mechanisms of power over life and death that modern society has established. For this reason, any minimization of racism is unacceptable, both for those who discriminate for the most futile reasons and for those who designate human lives as expendable in the name of balance and political compromises.

Faced with forms of racism, even apparently superficial, one must always keep one's guard high, because racism is not an ideology, it is simply a crime.

We must even be wary of the forced integration process. The emphasis on uncritical integration translates into specific control policy measures. For example, the introduction of compulsory language tests for migrants could become a subtle mechanism for keeping the immigrant under observation.

The emphasis with which the concrete implementation of the integration processes is expected, with increasing degrees, only creates the conditions for its incorrect application. The migrant is seen as a subject with a deficit and a cultural lack, therefore unreliable. He himself feels guilty, sentenced to exclusion for not doing something. He is completely dominated by the aggressiveness of an entire society, which had elected him as the scapegoat for his own survival.

Modern society is founded on the pervasiveness of the rules, to regulate the social behavior of citizens.

Racial Discrimination

The expression racial discrimination defines every action that without any justification disadvantages certain people, humiliates them, threatens them. Sometimes it endangers life, the physical, ethnic, cultural and religious integrity of the different.

Unlike racism, racial discrimination has no ideological motivation. It is the consequence of ignorance, widespread fears, prejudices and, in general, a lack of empathy.

The prevention and awareness work does not aim to identify racist subjects, as there is the risk of creating new scapegoats. The first step in the fight against racial discrimination is to recognize the suffering suffered by the victims of similar acts. Once it is admitted that racial discrimination exists on a structural, institutional and individual level, the only tools that allow us to fight it constantly are knowledge and culture. It is important to establish, in everyday life, the necessary conditions to avoid the occurrence of racial discrimination episodes.

Racial discrimination was legitimized in the modern age by the theoretical system of racism, by the cultural pride of all civilizations towards foreigners and by pride in the purity of blood.

In the States, these attitudes have given rise to two forms of discrimination, against women and against foreigners.

Discrimination against women resulted in slavery. The ancestors of today's African Americans were servants at least for the first generations. Their mulatto or black children were used as field slaves, they worked in worse conditions than the houseworkers.

In reality, all countries and all cultures have their own forms of racial discrimination, obvious or occult.

Racial discrimination exists whenever men of different races come into contact with each other and the strongest takes over the weakest.

Slavery

Slavery is the condition of one person completely subjected to another. Its role is to perform a task under the exclusive property of its owner. Slavery involves subjecting an individual to the will of the owner.

The exploration of Africa, the invasion of the Americas by Europeans in the fifteenth century and the subsequent colonization of these territories gave a great boost to the slave trade.

Portugal, which needed agricultural workers, was the first European state to use slaves to meet internal labor needs. Spain soon followed the Portuguese example.

In the same years, the African slave trade was also intensified by Arab traders. African slaves were believed to be better able to withstand very strenuous jobs such as the cultivation of sugar cane in tropical climates.

The number of African slaves grew enormously and it became fundamental for the economy and for the social system to find a legal formalization of their civil status.

Formally the slaves of America enjoyed certain rights, as in the case of private property. However, these were rights that the slave owner was not obliged to respect and in any case isolated cases. In general, basic human rights were in fact constantly violated.

Slaves could, for example, suffer sexual violence from their owners, families could be separated because their members were sold to different plantations. Brutal treatments such as mutilations and murders, theoretically prohibited by law, remained fairly common until the 19th century. Slave owners were then forbidden to teach them to read.

Racism against Blacks.

In racism against blacks, the hostility attitude is focused exclusively on a somatic trait: the color of the skin.

Discrimination against blacks was an essential element of the racist ideology that emerged during the 17th and 18th centuries. It was functional for the preservation of the colonial and slave system.

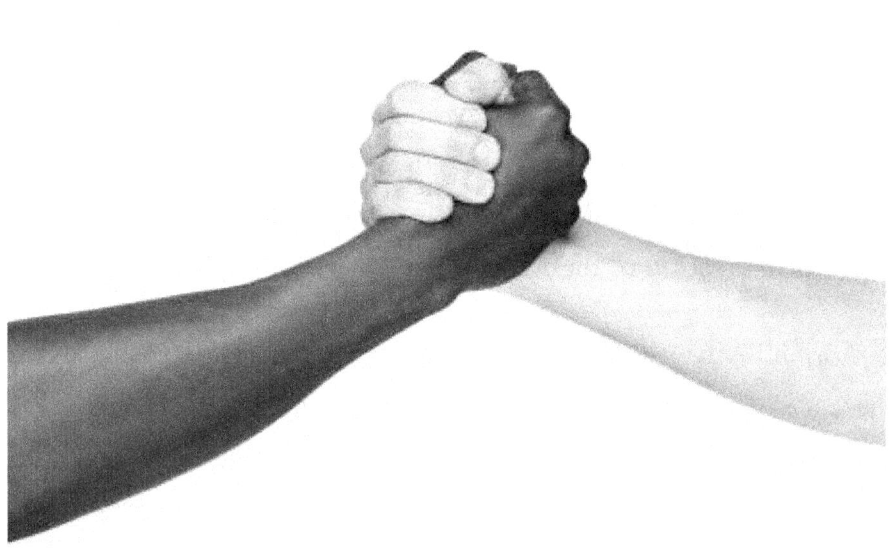

The European colonial powers legitimized slavery with religious references by arguing that blacks were morally and mentally backward. Blacks are associated with various negative behaviors such as forms of violence, illegal activities and exaggerated compotations.

All the British, French, Dutch, Spanish and Portuguese white elites exploited the slave labor of Africa systematically. In 1960 the United States eliminated slavery while in South Africa the apartheid regime was established, that is, racial segregation sanctioned by law and abolished in 1990.

Currently the forms and manifestations of racism against blacks are intensifying more and more. They range from daily and small-scale racism, to more subtle and hidden attitudes, up to the obvious rejection

Black people are often subject to this type of control which goes by the name of profiling. It occurs when a person is checked by the police force without concrete suspicion, solely for reasons related to the color of the skin.

The mechanism that triggers racism against blacks is due to clearly evident external characteristics. Unlike other minorities who base their diversity on religion or culture, less obvious from the color of the skin. This situation allows us to affirm, paradoxically, that blacks suffer double and frequent discrimination.

In the United States this is made even more blatant, because it boasts of being a great country, where national life is inspired by democratic ideals.

Different Forms of Racism.

Racism is based on the exaltation of biological differences such as the color of the skin, the shape of the body, the ways of posing and dressing and on the belief that the subjects in question belong to lower races. In different cultures there remains a strong sense of superiority towards others considered backward and far from an appreciable level of civilization.

These sensations derive, in general, from an incorrect perception of the different, from ignoring centuries of discrimination and exploitation. This way of behaving translates into a persistent hostility towards the different to defend one's identity.

Racism causes situations of marginalization towards minority ethnic groups and there is a tendency to divide society in us and them, in good and bad, in friends and enemies. The training received in the family, the culture of the community to which they belong and the influence of the mass media are the means to assimilate racist ideas. It is a kind of self-deception in its most masked forms which deludes the racists of their superiority.

In post-industrial and globalized society, racism presents itself even more as a very dangerous phenomenon. The distorted perception that it attributes to minorities, that is, negative behavior, criminal activities, such as prostitution and drug dealing, causes fears, systematically exploited by political propaganda and fueled by the mass media.

This type of racism arises from the desire to defend one's territory, from the fear of losing one's job and from the concern that urban ghettos marked by social degradation will form. It is a form of racism that could be defined as competitive. There is a sort of war between the local poor and foreigners.

Then there is cultural racism that arises from the desire to defend one's life system and culture, one's traditions and at the same time denigrates the values and culture of others. Subversive racism is linked to cultural racism. It manifests itself through a feeling of hostility towards all that is different. We try to avoid any contact with minorities, to limit the moments of interaction and to take all measures capable of keeping our distances, even going as far as real forms of segregation.

Finally, antithetical racism is based on the belief of a substantial irreconcilability between different cultures. It is considered necessary to safeguard its specificity, with a clear social and political closure towards minorities. Cultural diversity is not considered an enrichment factor, but an insurmountable barrier. Minorities are seen as enemies.

2.STEREOTYPES AND PREJUDICES.

Common Attitudes.

Stereotypes are the beliefs that we have about the characteristics of a group, while prejudices refer to the negative evaluation of the group.

The former arise from general knowledge of the group, the latter arise when we attribute these general characteristics to each member of the group. If stereotypes are normal and social, prejudices generally have an implicit negative connotation. An example of a stereotype is the belief that the inhabitants of the United States are all wealthy. While an example of prejudice is when we say that black people are violent and unreliable. This is discrimination.

They are large groups to which we attribute characteristics. The problem is when it leads to discrimination, which puts into practice the behavior aroused by both stereotype and prejudice. Stereotypes and prejudices play the role of simplifying reality. Maintaining some social control by forming groups makes it easier to maintain control of the world which is made more predictable.

The nature of stereotypes and prejudices is linked to the paths that the individual takes during his life and to the individual motivations that guide his actions. Each individual confronts different subjects and learns to evaluate himself in relation to others. It builds a large part of the self-image through the image of the group to which it belongs.

As one's personal identity and belonging to a society are formed, the self-esteem that the individual has of himself is natural. However, when you have an excess of self-esteem, you end up attributing successes only to your personal qualities and failures to external causes.

The individual is especially inclined to associate with people from whom he can have a confirmation of his ideas and image. He establishes a confrontation with the people from whom he obtains a positive judgment and refuses a confrontation with people who have different cultures and ideas.

In any case, stereotypes are the basis of prejudices, therefore limiting them will not become decisive for us. Changing a stereotype or prejudice is possible only if we approach the group and try to observe without filters and without wanting to confirm previously formulated opinions. Indeed, the point is precisely to dispel these ideas and dedicate our efforts to thoughts and situations that totally deviate from them. Our motto must be "we were all human beings, until religion separated us, politics divided us, and money classified us".

The National Characters.

There are certain stereotypes and prejudices that are based on the relevance given to national characters. The relative homogeneity of the national characters is determined by the socialization processes deriving from the family, the school and the mass media. These are characters based on simplified assessments of individual nationalities, based on particular characteristics extended to an entire nation. There is a possibility that an individual has some typical traits that contribute to forming the so-called national character. There is a generalization process that gives rise to stereotypes and prejudices capable of creating difficulties in relations between members of different national groups. Due to these approvals, individuals may be less available for constructive confrontation and interaction. They could show a fundamental hostility that does not predispose to overcoming cultural divergences and dialogue to facilitate civil coexistence.

Social Exclusion.

There are prejudices and stereotypes with a strong social impact. They have the ability to condition assessments towards other people, from whom we expect certain behaviors. When you are disappointed, you determine a formulation of negative judgments, even more so, towards them, of people with physical disabilities.

For centuries, the disabled have been the object of manifest hostility to the point of translating into forms of imprisonment. Some stereotypes have helped to consider physically disabled people as a category in themselves, made up of low-skilled and psychologically fragile subjects. Too emotional, unreliable, so we tend to show an embarrassment towards them that comes from not knowing how to behave.

Fortunately, in contemporary society, physical disability has been formally accepted and the social status of a protected category has been recognized, with advantages in terms of assistance and employment. Laws have been introduced that aim to hinder discrimination even if some stereotypes and prejudices remain.

Mental disability presents itself in a more complex way, because in addition to not meeting the efficiency standards established in society, it has always represented a mysterious and disturbing phenomenon.

Over the centuries a sense of repulsion has built up around the figure of the madman, accompanied by a magical-sacral reverence, as if the patient were in contact with supernatural forces.

This explains how in certain historical periods crazy people have been persecuted even with violence. Only since the nineteenth century has the principle been introduced that they must be considered as a patient in need of treatment.

Despite the progress made, the madman has remained a particular type of disabled person. His illness refers to the most hidden aspects of our personality. It evokes the possible prevalence of instincts over behaviors regulated by social norms. The madman represents the stereotype of the dangerousness of the mentally ill regardless of the damage that he could cause. The idea of unpredictable behavior continues to persist, capable of undermining the rules of coexistence.

A social phenomenon that has a serious negative impact is represented by drug addiction. Consumer subjects cause social damage resulting from the trade and sale of narcotic substances, almost always under the control of organized crime. It feeds petty crime and prostitution on the territory and manifests forms of family and individual violence.

This phenomenon of undoubted gravity often leads to considering the drug addict a subject with a fragile personality with high social danger. These negative assessments sometimes overshadow the multiple social, psychological, economic and environmental causes that determine drug addiction. They neglect the particular paths of life that have led an individual to fall into drug addiction.

Homophobia.

It is a stereotype based on fear and on an irrational form of aversion towards homosexuality, bisexuality and transsexuality. This attitude can be equated with racism and xenophobia in that it implies a set of feelings and behaviors adverse to different people.

The preliminary ruling regards homophobia as a socially and morally dangerous condition. It is therefore considered right to deny homosexual people social and legal recognition. Forms of discrimination in institutions, in cultural and artistic activities, in the workplace, up to forms of psychological repulsion are very often considered right. The psychopathological meaning considers aversion to homosexuals not only the result of negative prejudice, but is a phobia. An irrational and persistent fear and repugnance capable of compromising a person's psychological functioning.

Homophobia can be linked to a political ideology, to a specific cultural formation, to a religious condemnation, to a psychological imbalance on a personal level. All this leads to justify acts of violence or discrimination against people because of a real or presumed homosexuality.

It has been found that authoritarian or insecure people who feel threatened by someone other than themselves tend to homophobia, or are struggling with a strong latent and repressed homosexuality.

Xenophobia.

Xenophobia (from the Greek "fear of the foreigner"). Although they may share some characteristics, xenophobia and racism are nevertheless different phenomena. Racism conceives the immigrant as belonging to an inferior race, xenophobia as a threat. Xenophobia is based on an idea of national superiority and which sees foreigners as a threat, because it belongs to another type of society.

Xenophobia arises and spreads when the foreigner is somehow internal to his world, when he creates the feeling of being an invader. It provokes the conviction that we must remove, discriminate, marginalize the sanier, or wage war to exterminate him.

Manifested by his physical appearance, cultural traits, ways and language of origin, the foreigner is seen as an inferior individual. On the contrary, the natives are those born and rooted in the territory where they live. From this spatial location they derive the feeling of their superiority towards the foreigner.

Xenophobia is an attitude based on prejudices and stereotypes that associates negative feelings with everything that is considered foreign. The construction of images of alleged foreigners does not have anthropological, but socio-cultural reasons. In other words, it is not given by nature and can therefore be changed.

Xenophobia can be caused by the fear, by the natives, of a social descent, by anxieties of status and by a lack of confidence in the ability to affirm one's own cultural identity.

Normally the fear of the foreigner rarely occurs in a pure state, it can be accompanied by a certain interest and curiosity. These feelings coexist, mix according to varying proportions and it rarely happens that one prevails over the other. For this reason, the encounter between foreigners and natives is dominated by a substantial ambivalence, the foreigner can be admired or despised.

Sociology has found that relations between the foreigner and the members of the host society are characterized primarily by ambivalence. Society marginalizes the foreigner but at the same time needs it to feed its economy, to fulfill those tasks that the natives reject, occupying places that would otherwise be free.

To eliminate ambivalence and the possible onset of xenophobia, it is useful to strengthen intercultural communication relationships. It must be taken into account that it is certainly difficult for the foreigner to integrate with the cultural and community institutions and traditions in which he has joined. His first goal is to get that job and achieve the well-being that would be barred from him at home.

If he does not obtain citizenship, he can exercise a limited influence on the processes of cultural change, because the contact between two different cultures produces significant social changes quite slowly.

When major social and economic changes occur that cause unemployment, strong migratory flows and political power focuses on nationalism, insecure and fear, intercultural communication processes can be interrupted. In any case, a strong emotional reaction is generated which manifests itself as a desire for rejection and destruction which results in xenophobia.

Right-wing extremism is based on the belief that humans are not all the same. An ideology of exclusion that can go hand in hand with a high degree of acceptance of violence.

All the definitions of right-wing extremism agree in identifying its constituent components in racism and xenophobia. Right-wing extremists believe that social inequalities are due to racial or ethnic factors. Human rights are not considered valid principles everywhere, therefore the multiculturalism of globalized society must be rejected and combated.

To enhance the development of one's identity, however, contact with different cultures based on intellectual curiosity and the desire for comparison would be useful. To do this, it is necessary to be aware that there is no perfect cultural identity. Cultures are heterogeneous and changing constructions, subjected to continuous processes of contamination by other cultures. In this perspective, the foreigner must not be seen as someone who invades your territory, but a person who must be welcomed, for the development of cultural life and society.

Different Discrimination

Direct discrimination occurs if a person suffers a difference in treatment due only to his belonging to a group that in the past has tended to be marginalized or treated as inferior and still is.

If expressed privately, racial personal opinions are protected by freedom of expression and are not legally punishable. Racist attitudes do not necessarily result in racist acts and do not necessarily have an ideological foundation. However, they can contribute to a climate in which racist claims and discriminatory acts are more easily tolerated or approved, even if they remain unrelated to the practice of the majority of the population.

Direct discrimination occurs when a person, for inadmissible reasons, is at a disadvantage compared to another who is in a similar situation. A person is disadvantaged, solely because of a distinctive feature of his identity. Discrimination therefore also affects aspects of human dignity. Indirect discrimination occurs when, despite their apparent neutrality, legal, political or practical bases result in unequal treatment.

Multiple discrimination occurs when a person is discriminated against at the same time due to multiple characteristics, physiognomic characteristics or religious affiliation and sex, social class and a disability.

In the case of intersectional discrimination, however, different forms of exclusion interact in such a way as to highlight one in particular. For example, racist behavior towards a woman can manifest itself in the form of sexism or, on the contrary, an act that is actually sexist in nature can be motivated with racist arguments.

Anti-Muslim Hostility.

The term anti-Muslim hostility designates an attitude of rejection towards people who define themselves as Muslims or are perceived as such. In anti-Muslim hostility, elements of refusal can flow towards people originating from certain countries, from companies considered patriarchal or from the fundamentalist practice of faith.

The belief that all Muslims want to introduce sharia, do not respect human rights and sympathize with terrorists also falls within the vision of anti-Muslims.

The term "anti-Muslim hostility" is preferred to the term "Islamophobia", as state measures against discrimination against

Muslims are intended to protect individuals and groups of individuals, not a religion.

The use of the term Islamophobia hides risks, as it explains the processes of stigmatization in psychological and biological terms, thus suggesting that violence and exclusion are given by nature.

Anti-Semitism / Anti-Jewish Hostility.

The term "anti-Jewish hostility" means an attitude of rejection towards people who define themselves as Jewish or are perceived as such. The term anti-Semitism is used today as a synonym for all anti-Jewish attitudes. Anti-Semitism is a particular form of racism in which an ethnic belonging is matched to a religious belonging.

Anti-Semitism includes racist offenses, such as attacks on the physical integrity or property of Jews and Jewish institutions. Together with the legal means offered by civil law, the prosecution of anti-Jewish or anti-Semitic crimes constitute important elements of the necessary measures against anti-Semitism.

On the other hand, they can also be clearly or vaguely recognizable prejudices or stereotypes to put one's own group before that of the Jews or to denigrate or disadvantage the Jews and their institutions.

State measures against discrimination against Jews or people perceived as such are intended to protect individuals and groups of individuals, not a religion. Measures must therefore be taken in all social spheres and at all institutional levels, and especially at the individual level.

Gypsyism.

Anti-Gypsyism is a concept coined in analogy to anti-Semitism and in use since the 1980s. The hostile attitude towards people or groups of people perceived as Gypsies is designated, regardless of whether they lead a nomadic life or not.

Throughout history, anti-Gypsyism has manifested itself in the form of economic and social discrimination. It has reached the point of political persecution, internment, forced sterilization and genocide organized by the state apparatus. The term Gypsy is conceived by many as a racist connotation, because it spreads negative content even if it is used in reference to hostility towards the Jenisch, Sinti and Roma.

3. RACISM IN AMERICA

Historical Summary.

The term race, from which racism derives, is of uncertain origin and was introduced into European languages around the 16th century. It was used in John Fox's Book of Martyrs (1563) to indicate the race, in this case the race of Abraham.

From the 16th century onwards, to explain the differences between Africans, Chinese and Europeans, instead of the term races, the genealogies of the different ethnic groups described in the Old Testament were used. At the end of the seventeenth century, the debate developed on the morality of the slave trade between one side of the Atlantic and the other. The debate began between those in favor and those opposed to slavery. For the first time it was pointed out that blacks and whites shared a common humanity.

The term race returned to be used in relation to the relative technological backwardness of Africans, which was considered the result of their unhealthy living conditions, due both to the climate and to the lack of political and social institutions that promoted their progress. These behaviors were the basis of attempts to legitimize discrimination first and then slavery.

Although Charles Darwin's book "The origin of the species" (1859), which documented how development was produced by natural selection, revolutionized theories of differences between humans in science, it did not prevent a distorted use of the term race. Indeed, it inspired a new form of racism, the so-called scientific racism, based on the idea that racial prejudice even performs an evolutionary function.

The sociological theory of racism dates back to the early 1920s when some psychologists began to argue that racial prejudice was not a hereditary feature but a form of behavior learned during socialization.

Each society has its own culture and, at the same time, is subject to a series of cultural prejudices. Ethnocentrism, the tendency to make judgments as if one's culture and ethnic group were at the center of the world, is responsible for this way of reasoning.

The Causes of Racism.

Racism can be a consequence of migratory phenomena, especially if generally due to economic reasons and the lack of job opportunities in the regions of origin. In these cases, immigration is perceived as a threat to the well-being of local populations, who develop a feeling of intolerance and distrust of new arrivals. We are faced with real xenophobia.

In the 1960s, the spread of the practice of intelligence tests rekindled the controversy about the inheritance of intelligence in the scientific world. More than anything else, it was better to refer to that particular concept of intelligence detected by the tests of the intelligence quotient, IQ. New impetus was given to forms of racism based on the alleged inferiority of some ethnic groups.

However, scientifically proving how a characteristic is a product of inheritance or a consequence of socialization is nevertheless extremely difficult. In fact, those who supported the first hypothesis were accused of encouraging a new scientific racism.

The linguist William Labov has in fact documented, thanks to numerous researches, how tests build intelligence rather than measure it. In his article, "Black Intelligence and Academic Ignorance" argued that intelligence tests are ethnocentric because they are based on a restricted concept of intelligence.

According to the linguist, it was only a matter of supporting logical operations, typical of western culture, in which it is obvious that whites are more skilled on average, at least in the short term. The test results would therefore have nothing to do with genetic differences but would only reflect the ethnocentric way in which the test is formulated.

The Integration Process.

The racially based caste-based society pattern of Spanish-American colonies extended to British colonies in North America with the arrival of the first black slaves in Jamestown (Virginia) in 1619. This event had historical and explosiveconsequences, the effects of which continue to this day. The United States subsequently maintained slavery as an institution, despite the country's profoundly democratic inspiration, it had a racially divided society.

The abolition of slavery, implemented first in the Northern States with a gradual process which ended in 1827, and then in those of the South after the civil war (1861-1865), had two consequences. In the first place racial discrimination soon followed slavery, then with a slower process, under the pressure of progressive industrialization, society divided into racially based castes became a society divided into social classes.

The breed, recognizable by the color of its skin and other characteristics, remained equally important for the social position of individuals and groups. The racial barriers existing between the castes became more permeable to a greater social rise.

On the other hand, the white rulers tried in every way to prevent blacks from any socio-economic improvement with unfavorable laws. Social pressures then followed up to the extreme case of the Ku Klux Klan. The blacks were to be kept in their places, possibly relegated forever to the lower end of the social pyramid.

In 1770, that is, even before independence, slavery was prohibited for the first time in Maine, at the northeastern end of the future United States. At the same time in this region, where no African American lived then, immigration of blacks was prohibited.

In 1787, when the Constituent Assembly met in Philadelphia, which was at that time the most populous city of the young Confederation and its temporary capital, the Southern States, threatening a secession, asserted their sovereign right to the maintenance of slavery in their territories.

Simultaneously in the same city racial discrimination began against black members in the ecclesiastical environment, even in the Methodist Church, which tended to be democratic.

In protest, the initial nucleus of what would become the first African American Church, the African Methodist Episcopal Church, was formed. However, in 1827, the year of the abolition of slavery, black people in Philadelphia began to be openly discriminated against in the use of the first means of mass public transport, born from industrialization.

African Americans with bitterness in their grievances, noticed that this was happening in the same city that took its name from fraternal love and that had contributed so much to the education and emancipation of blacks.

The dialectical relationship between emancipation and racial discrimination continued to exist even after the civil war, which had as its cause the question of slavery and as a more important result its abolition in the defeated South.

After the confused interlude of the so-called, era of reconstruction, (1865-1877), most of the liberal abolitionists of the North tolerated the movement for the exclusion of African Americans from civil rights in the already slave states .From

1890 onwards the constitutions of the individual southern states, starting with the southern ones, sanctioned this exclusion.

By 1910, New South's racial discrimination regime was consolidated everywhere, destined to survive almost entirely for half a century. The same happened with the suppression of administrative autonomy in Washington, the federal capital, decided in 1883 after the number of African American inhabitants exceeded that of whites.

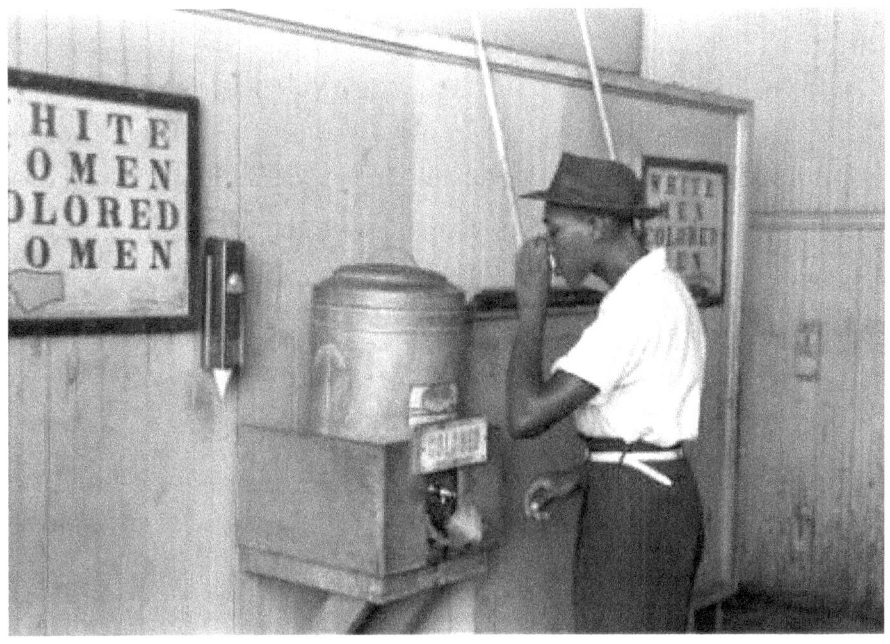

Against the division of American society into a society for whites and a society for blacks, the idea of racial integration developed. Discrimination had to be accepted as a temporary phenomenon and then overcome in the long term through an autonomous process of industrialization, conducted by the same black population. It was believed that defeating racial discrimination following the abolition of slavery could only be overcome. The blacks would become an active component of the economy on their own and would also organize themselves politically in American democratic society.

There were those who focused on intellectual education, for the integration of blacks, and consequently for the formation of a future elite of color. Acting, so to speak, from above, in connection with white philanthropists, mostly Jews, who would have supported such ideas to achieve democracy in the United States, it was intended to be achieved peacefully.

A Brief History of the Indian Wars in the USA.

Between the seventeenth and nineteenth centuries, the natives of North America waged wars to stop the expansionism of European colonists in an attempt to prevent their settlement on their territories.

The divisions existing between the Indian nations and the inadequacy of the means at their disposal reduced the clash to a long series of defeats and massacres of the natives, interrupted by victories that immediately became a legend precisely because of their exceptional nature.

In the early nineteenth century the Shawnee chief Tecumseh managed to organize a confederation of Indian nations that alarmed the governor of the Indiana Territory, who resumed hostilities and in the battle of Tippecanoe defeated the confederation.

Whole Indian nations were expelled from their territories of origin and deported to the west of Mississippi: Sauk, Fox, Creek, Cherokee, tried in vain to resist, but by the end of the 1950s all Indian presence in the eastern part of the United States had effectively disappeared.

Between 1840 and 1890, the federal government organized a system of reserves within which to force Indian nations, thus initiating the conquest and colonization of the western territories. In the mid-century Bannock and Shoshone from Oregon and Idaho, Utes from Nevada and Utah, Apaches and Navajo from the southeastern territories joined forces in a vast but ineffective attempt at rebellion.

Between the 1860s and 1870s Arapaho, Cheyenne and Sioux waged a war fought with particular ferocity on both sides, during which the mythical battle of Little Bighorn took place (June 25, 1876), during which the VII Cavalry Regiment led by General Custer was annihilated by Cheyenne and Sioux of Sitting Bull and Crazy Horse, both of whom were forced to surrender within a year.

The last extensive action of resistance was conducted by the Apaches of Geronimo. On 29 December 1890 with the Wounded Knee massacre in South Dakota, where the Federal Cavalry massacred Sioux men, women and children, the Indian wars ended.

Ku Klux Klan.

It is a secret terrorist organization, founded in 1866 in Pulaski, Tennessee, after the Secession war. Assertors of the inferiority of blacks, and therefore of the inopportunity to recognize their civil and political rights.

Covered in white tunics and masked by long pointed hoods, the Klansmen began to terrorize the more enterprising blacks so that they did not exercise the newly acquired political rights, nor did they carry out public activity. The threats were followed by floggings and mutilations, up to the assassination.

The criminal activity pushed the government to decree the dissolution of the Klan. In 1870 the name, rituals and attitudes of the original Klan reappeared in a new organization, the Invisible Empire, Knights of the Ku Klux Klan, founded in 1915 in Georgia.

In addition to African Americans, Catholics and Jews also became subject to Klan intimidation. The wave of violence peaked in the 1920s, especially in the southern states. In the years of the Great Depression, a downsizing followed, until the dissolution of the Invisible Empire in 1944.

With the strengthening of the movement for civil rights of the fifties and sixties, the Klan attempted the revival by proposing itself as an advanced and radical point of the front of opposition to racial integration. At the end of the eighties it was made up of about fifteen organizations, with an overall follow-up estimated at around 5000 units.

The First Black Organizations.

In the 1877 compromise, the political leaders of the north withdrew the federal troops of the southern states, at the same time the police state began in the south.

Between 1890 and 1905 the south enacted the complex of segregationist laws. Booker T. Washington organizes the National negro Business League in Boston, aimed at developing the black bourgeoisie.

In 1905 W.E.B Du Bois founded the Niagara Movement, the first expression of the black movement, as opposed to the organization of B.T. Washington. The Niagara Movement broke up four years later, while a group of whites organized the National Negro Committee.

In 1911 some whites founded the NUL, National Urban League, for the inclusion of Negroes in industrial production. Two years later in Newark, Noble Drew Ali founded the Moorisch American Science Temple, while Carter G. Woodson founded the Association for the Study of Negro Life and History. A very important date was 1917 when Marcus Garvery founded the Unia, Universal Negro Improvement Association. for the separation between Negroes and whites and for the "return" of Negroes to Africa. It will have up to 3 million members and, during the First World War, it will become the first popular Negro movement with mass characteristics.

In 1919 the Commission on Interrracial Cooperation was born, which in 1944 was transformed into the Southern Regional

Council, to reconcile the contrasts that exploded in the South when the veterans of the World War I claimed to "boast" the ribbons of veterans.

Twelve years later W. Dard founded the Nation of Islam (Black Muslims) and appoints his first pastor Elijah Muhammad, who in 1934 will become head of the sect. In 1933 the Southern Conference for Human Welfare was born, whose educational sector will become autonomous with the name of SCEF (Southern Conference Educational Fund).

The National Negro Congress was founded in 1935, an organization aimed at uniting all the trade unions and black associations. A.Philip Randolph, president of the League of sleeping bag wagons, takes over the presidency. In 1940 the majority of members joined the PC and Randolph resigned. After a year in January, Randolph proposes a Negro march on Washington; The Movement of Washington March against discrimination in the war industries was born.

The Racial Explosion in the Post-War Period.

Between 1940 and 1960, Negroes residing outside the 11 states of the old confederation increased more than double, that is, more than less than 4 million in 1940 to more than 9 million in 1960, roughly half of the entire Negro population in the USA.

Much of this increase was concentrated in the 12 largest cities in the US, which now house between a quarter and a third of all black Americans. In the cities of Washington and New York, Negroes represent the majority of the population. In Detroit,

Baltimore, Cleveland and St Louis, they make up more than a third and in many other cities such as Chicago, Philadelphia, Cincinnati, Indianapolis and Oakland they far exceed the fourth part. In 1943 CORE, Congress of Racial Equality was founded.

After the Nazi aggression to the USSR, the major black organizations agreed on the desirability of blacks enlisting. Their number rises from 115,197 in 1941 to 1,174,000. In addition, about a million Negroes are engaged in the war industries.

In February 1960, in a bar in Greensboro, four black university students were refused a coffee they had asked for, continued to remain seated, and thus the idea of sit-in was born. Over 90 white and black students will have completed it in May.

On the eve of Easter in Raleigh the 1st conference of students from the south is held, organized by the SCLC. The SNCC, Student Nonviolent Coordinating Committee is born. CORE organizes the first Freedom Rides to abolish segregation in the waiting rooms of southern public transport. The slogan "throw your body into the fight" spreads.

In the summer, a group of SNCC leaders travel to Jackson and organize support for Freedom Rides. Towards the end of the year, a period of sit-ins, marches, mass arrests begins in Albany. On April 27, 1962, police raided the mosque of the Nation of Islam in Los Angeles, kill a Negro and injure 11 others.

It was reconstituted after a long inactivity, the SDS, Students for A Democratic Society, and the NSM, Northern Student

Movement were founded. Together with the SNCC, they form radical student organizations.

The following year there was a riot in the Birmingham ghetto. The premises were created by the Alabama Christian Movement for Human Rights, made up of poor Negroes. The unrest spread to 30 cities. Kennedy is forced to announce new civil rights legislation. In August, 250,000 demonstrators march on Washington to gain full recognition of civil rights. The march is carried out by leader Bayard Rustin and supported by all associations.

The Chicago Uprising reaches its peak in the fall. The premise dates back to 1960, i.e. the formation of TWO, the Woodlawn Residents Organization. It was the first successful attempt to mobilize neighborhood blacks in a single organization. The TWO, in fact, was born from the merger of over 90 groups of different nature. There are serious racial incidents in Birmingham. 5 Negroes are killed in Mississippi during the year. In 1964, the civil rights law passed by Kennedy was approved.

The "Summer Project" was launched in Mississippi, the first Negro electoral group outside the Democratic Party, sending its delegates to the Atlantic City convention in August with a petition calling for representation of the state of Mississippi.

The Cleveland conference was held on February 19, 1965, in which 150 poor whites and blacks from various northern cities set out the positions of their groupings. In March, a march takes place from Selma to Montogomery, for 5 days, 30,000 people protest against the non-registration of blacks on the southern electoral lists; in August, Johnson is forced to guarantee the right to vote for southern blacks.

From 12 to 19 August, riot in the Watts ghetto: 34 Negroes killed. In April, the Lowndes County Freedom Organization formed a party to present black candidates for elections in Lowndes County; a black panther is chosen as the electoral symbol. The first issue of the BPP weekly, "The Black Panthers", was released in April. In 1969 in Los Angeles, 2 panthers were assassinated by Ron Karenga's nationalist black organization. On April 3 of the same year, 21 panthers were arrested in New York; they are suspected of having organized a plan for attacks on radio stations, department stores, etc. These acts of violence will be repeated very frequently in the largest American cities. In September 1970 the 1st BPP Congress took place in Philadelphia.

The Current Situation.

Many problems in the African American community persist. The current average income of a black family is only three-fifths of that of a white family. Social integration, still incomplete, has ended up reviving the supporters of a desirable "separation" of black society and culture from white ones. Obviously to be expressed not necessarily in conflicting forms, but certainly with a strong emphasis on one's originality and diversity.

This growing trend towards a dichotomy is evident above all in the field of culture and the arts, from rap music to the cinematography of Gordon Parks, Melvin Van Peebles or Spike

Lee, to the academic enhancement of African and African American history and traditions.

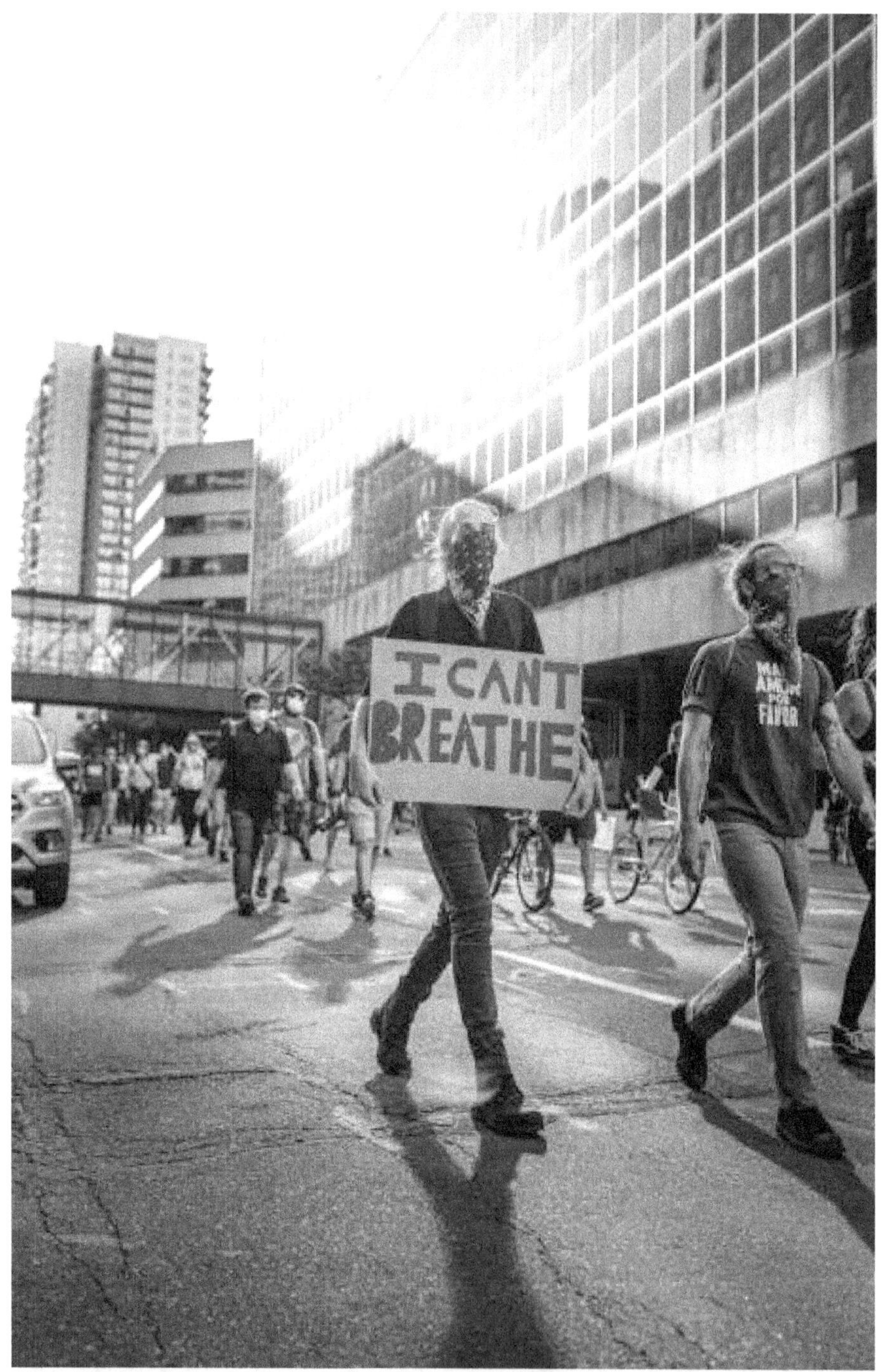

The common element is represented by the emphasis of the specificity of the contribution of black reality to an American culture in which the multiculturalism that had supported the myth of the melting pot in the sixties and seventies appears to have definitively entered into crisis.

4.HISTORICAL LEADERS

Marcus A. Garvey

The idea of racial integration found an opponent in Marcus A. Garvey (1870-1940), a Jamaican black, who starting in 1916 denounced American society as divided into racially based caste and classes and pointed to the blacks of integration as traitors.

Garvey appealed directly to black-skinned African Americans and their race pride, heirs to the field slaves. This led to making African Americans a caste in itself, a voluntarily segregated sub-company, endowed with specific structures not only political and social, but also economic and religious. He founded the new African Orthodox Church. He secretly accepted the financial and political support of white racist extremism on the Ku Klux Klan genre, and also sought to create an African American mass movement inspired by the old idea of "back to Africa".

Despite his political and organizational failure since 1923, Garvey left a deep footprint in the political consciousness of black Americans and young African nationalism, if only in English-speaking countries. When Ghana gained independence, it inserted the same red, green and black colors into its flag as those adopted by the Garvey movement. But in the final analysis, as its founder already pointed out, this movement resolved itself into a black racism which was opposed to the predominant one of whites, simply reversing their values, black is beautiful, white is ugly.

Malcolm X

America had to wait for a black president, capable of speaking to Islam, raised as a child in the shadow of the Jakarta minarets, then Harvard star, the statesman who dares to think of a pacified and post-racial society.

Only in the Barack Obama era does it become possible to reopen a great taboo, a page of tearing history. It is the story of Malcolm X, who died at the age of 39, hit by shots while haranguing the crowd in Harlem's Audubon Ballroom.

On February 21, 1965, on the day of a violent death that he himself had foreseen and announced, Malcolm X took many secrets to his grave, starting with the identity of his assassins and principals.

An extraordinary speaker, it became the screen on which millions of blacks projected their hopes. He had a lot of jazz improvisers, anticipated future rappers. It embodied the myth of the avenging outlaw, in a society of blacks without rights. He has been described as an artist who reinvents himself. He went from provincial offender to showman, from self-taught intellectual to radical exponent of black nationalism, religious preacher, Orthodox Muslim.

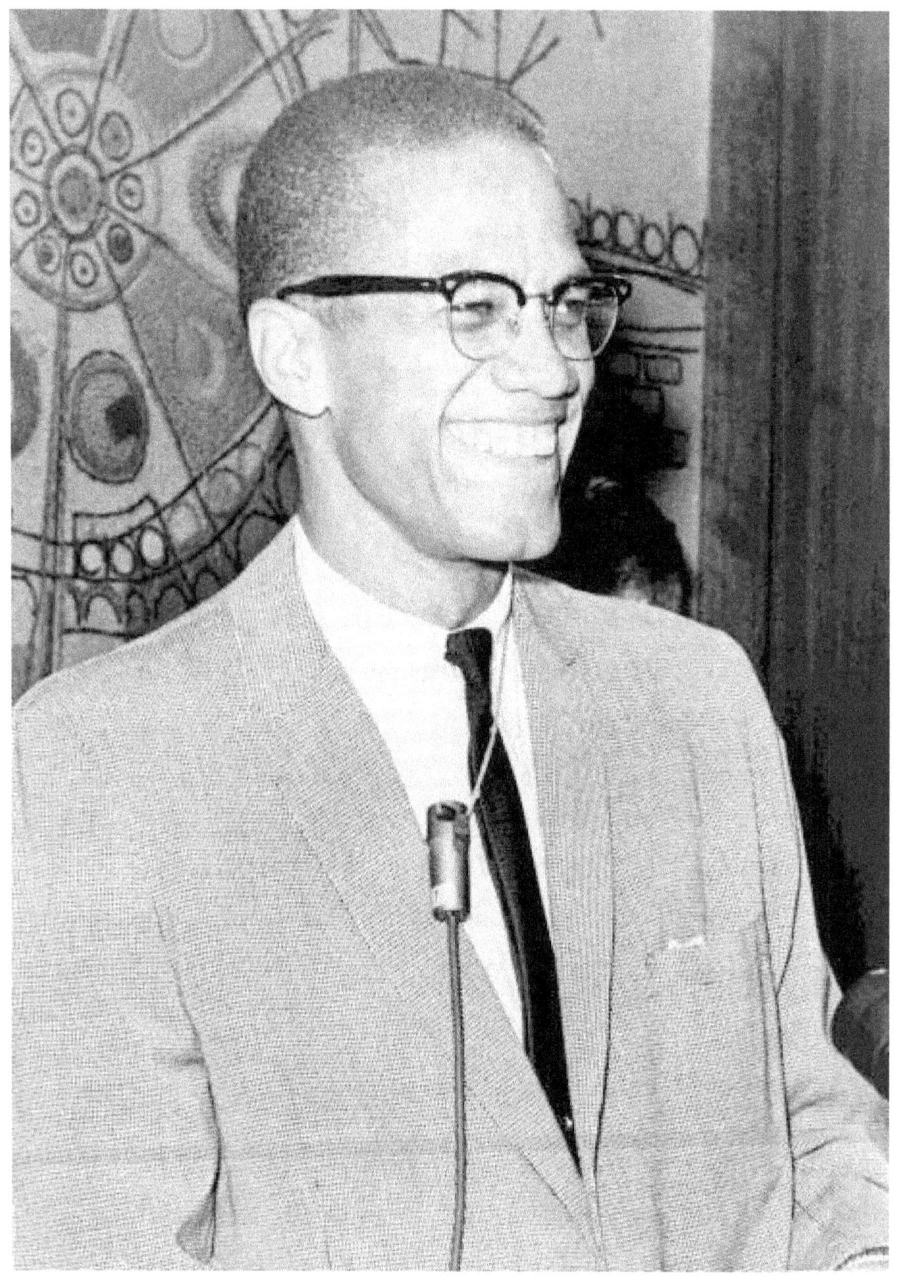

A bitter rival to Martin Luther King, then on the verge of being reconciled with him. One of the reasons for his early death. After the assassination of Malcolm X three men are arrested, tried, quickly convicted. Two will be released in the 1980s and have never stopped claiming to be innocent. Only the third, TalmadgeHayer, released from prison, is self-confessed.

It wasn't just him shooting that day. A meticulous investigation reconstructs a different truth. It was a commando of five hit men who signed the execution. Who fired the first shot, mortal, has never been disturbed by justice. Under the name William Bradley he was a former basketball champion, celebrated in the Newark Athletic Wall of Fame. The track of the principals forks in two opposite directions but equally interested in killing MalcolmX and then burying it in the porthole.

On the one hand there is the FBI which systematically intercepted his telephone calls, ignored the multiplying death threats, did everything to ensure that the attack proceeded undisturbed. On the other hand is black radicalism, starting with the Nation of Islam.

There is a lot of evidence accumulated about the killers and the principals, but reopening the investigation and doing justice today, going up the chain of command will never happen, because nobody wants it.

In Islam the young Malcolm Little of Omaha, Nebraska, arrives after numerous reincarnations, marked by changes of identity: Jack Carlton, Detroit Red (when he dyes his hair), Satan, El-Hajj Malik El-Shabazz. Finally, the X, symbol of rebellion against surnames that had been given to the slaves by the white masters. The son of a Baptist pastor who may have been murdered by whites himself, Malcolm grows up in such a poor family that often his mother can cook street weeds at dinner.

Become a drug dealer, then gang leader of thieves, in Detroit and Harlem. In prison for robbery from 1946 to 1952, at the Norfolk Prison Colony of Massachusetts. Here he converts to Islam, quits smoking and gambling, studies the history of African Americans and together Herodotus, Kant, Nietzsche. There the transition takes place between two equally popular roles in black mythology: the ruthless bandit avenger of the oppressed, and the preacher called to save their souls.

At the height of his fame Malcolm becomes the spokesman for the Nation of Islam and contributes to widening its ranks up to 500,000 members. It is the period of its extreme radicalization. When 62 wealthy Atlanta whites die in a plane crash, it is proof that God exists. Reacts to the assassination of John Kennedy by saying that he deserved it. He recruits in prisons, creating a total mix of political militancy and crime. Invoke armed struggle, defend terrorism against the police, become the theoretical precursor of the Black Panther.

Imagine a black nation seceding into America, to the point of meeting with exponents of the Ku Klux Klan to plan together the separation between the two races. The Nation of Islam, with Malcolm X, becomes a bizarre mix of theology, science fiction, racial fanaticism. Theorizes the intrinsic wickedness of the white race and in particular of the Jews, the inferiority of women. Divorce suddenly matures. For personal reasons too. The spiritual leader of the Nation of Islam, Elijah Muhammad, gets pregnant the woman with whom Malcolm had had a long relationship. And then there is the trip to Mecca, the encounter with a moderate and multiracial Islam. Another conversion to the Sunni faith. It is treason that arms his assassins.

Just when Malcolm begins to recover the dialogue with Martin Luther King, hitherto painted as an "uncle Tom", a silly servant of the whites. Malcolm had dismissively said against Martin Luther King: "There are more important things than the right to sit together with whites in a restaurant."

For the black poet Amiri Baraka he was not wrong, Malcolm X, and his legacy is less negative than it seems. Sense of identity, independence, with the values of the hard wing of the black liberation movement, had a huge impact on American society, without him there would be no Obama.

Here too, blacks continue to divide. Between those who see Malcolm as the champion of a race pride, and those who trace permanent victimhood to him. The angry black label that Obama managed to take off with enormous effort, stoically enduring the silly accusations about his Kenyan nationality or his alleged Islamic religion. And when in July 2009 Obama took up the defense of a Harvard black professor, Henry Louis Gates, who was subjected to police abuse, right - thinking and conservative white America jumped on Obama. Hoping he would react with nerves. Dreaming of finding a Malcolm X as an opponent: a Satan.

Martin Luther King

Less than forty years ago there were separate public drinking fountains for whites and blacks in the States. Thinking of Martin

Luther King, other famous examples come to mind, such as the separate balcony for blacks at the theater and the seats at the end of the bus only for blacks.

Hard to believe, but it was really not long ago. The struggle to change these conditions and gain equal rights before citizens of any ethnicity was the background to Martin Luther King's short life.

The pioneer Protestant pastor of the African American civil rights struggle was born on January 15, 1929 in Atlanta in the United States. At six he began attending school at Yonge Street Elementary School, after he had been expelled the year before because he was found to be taking courses at five.

His father, Martin Luther King senior, is a pastor of the Baptist Church, his mother a teacher. In very early childhood, little Martin used to play with white neighborhood children but, with the beginning of elementary school, some incomprehensible facts happened: he was excluded from the games of his neighbors and, even, children were strictly forbidden to speak with him.

Martin can't make up for it. Mum tries to cheer him up by talking to him about what it means to be black and live in a Southern state. She tells him about the distant African origins, the long and terrible slavery endured by his people, the Secession War that gave them, at least formally, the freedom.

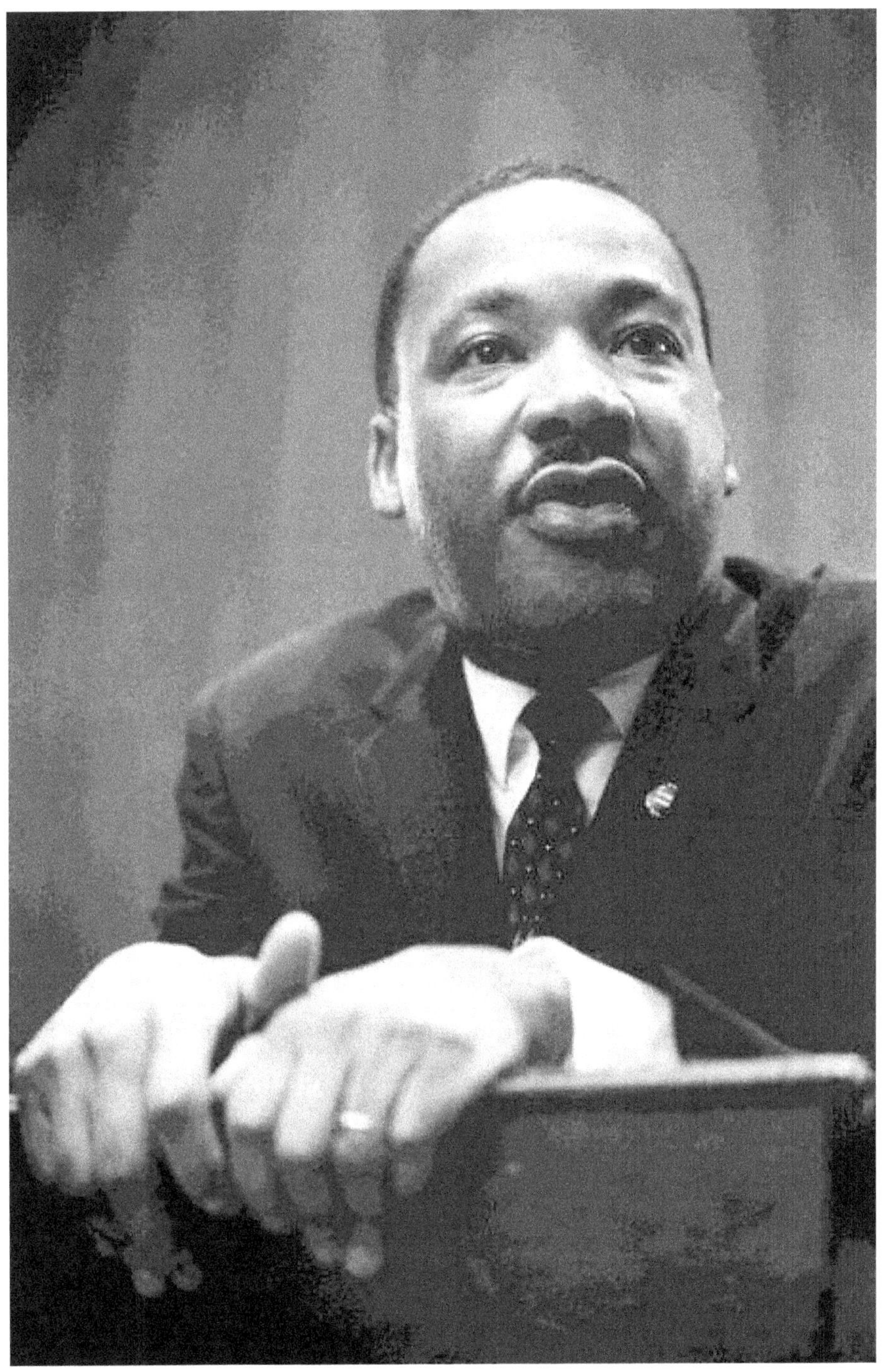

During his adolescence, while attending Morehouse College
thanks to a teacher, he understands the importance of religion.

Only faith in God allows black brothers to survive and believe that someone loves them up there. For the young man, this sentence is such a revelation that, after high school, he enrolled in the seminary in Chester, Pennsylvania. He completed his studies and, during the preparation of his graduation thesis (obtained later, at the University of Boston), he met a girl, Coretta Scott Young, who studied singing at the New England Conservatory with the hope of becoming soprano.

The woman comes from a family of modest origins (her father is a carpenter) who has in the past been subjected to harassment by some racist sects; Coretta also has the dream of being able to do something for her people.

The two young people fall in love and in 1953 they marry in Marion, the hometown of the young woman, and then move to Montgomery (Alabama) in the Southern States, where racial intolerance was greater: both are determined to fight to no longer be judged inferior, but be treated as citizens like the others. The model of struggle that inspires Martin Luther King's theory is that proposed by Mahatma Gandhi: non-violence. The question that always arose was to contrast the idea that a human being could be despised for the different color of their skin.

His sermons begin to make him famous among his brothers and not only. His battle for civil rights begins to attract more and more proselytes. In December 1955, an apparently trivial fact made a turning point in King's struggle. A black worker gets on a bus to go home. She worked all day and being very tired, she looks for a place to sit. Since all the seats reserved for blacks are occupied, she sits on one, among the many left free, reserved for whites. Rosa Parks' gesture is the classic drop that made the vase overflow. King calls a meeting of all his followers tired of being subjected to abuse, even worse than that suffered by the worker.

On this occasion the idea of boycotting all public transport is launched. No black man will get on the bus until the division of seats is removed. The initiative is hugely successful. The next day the public cars are completely empty, not only the blacks but also the whites join the non-violent struggle.

The situation continues, unchanged even in the following days, public transport remains empty. The authorities do not give up and, not knowing how to resolve the matter, sue Martin L. King for having damaged the public transport company. But when the process is about to start, great news comes. the United States Supreme Court has declared segregation practiced in buses illegal.

It's a huge victory for King, but its price is equally high. A charge of dynamite explodes in front of his house, he himself is stoned, beaten and attacked by the dogs of the national guard. He is also arrested about twenty times during the peace demonstrations and, more than once, John Kennedy himself, not yet elected president, personally pays the bail to get him out of prison.

In August 1963 Martin Luther King led a huge interracial demonstration in Washington, where he delivered a speech that touched the heart of the nation and millions of people took action. It combines the criteria of non-violence and Christian ones, and which begins with the words I have a dream… .. The following year he was awarded the Nobel Peace Prize and Pope Paul VI received him at the Vatican.

Unfortunately, however, the slowness of public powers and the constant and profound racism of whites, not only in the southern states, continues to exacerbate blacks who are increasingly choosing extremist solutions. In April 1968 he went to Memphis to participate in a march in favor of the city scavengers, black and white, who were on strike.

While on the veranda of the hotel, he talks to his collaborators, some rifle shots are fired from the house opposite: Martin Luther King falls on the railing. He will die a few minutes later. Taking advantage of the panic moments that follow, the killer vanishes.

It is 7pm on April 4, 1968. The killer will be arrested in London about two months later. His name is James Earl Ray, but he reveals that he was not Martin Luther King's killer. In fact, he claims to know who the real culprit is. Name he can never do because he will be stabbed the next night in his cell. Even today the mystery remains unsolved. Some argue that there are too many similarities between the King case and the Kennedy case to deal with mere coincidences. However, the culprits, if they are still alive, continue to be unknown.

Bayard Rustin

He was an organizer and civil rights activist, best known for his work as a consultant to Martin Luther King Jr. in the 1950s and 1960s.

Bayard Rustin was born in West Chester, Pennsylvania on March 17, 1912. He moved to New York in the 1930s and was involved in pacifist groups and early civil rights protests. Combining non-violent resistance with organizational skills, he was a key adviser to Martin Luther King Jr. in the 1960s. Although he has been arrested multiple times for his civil disobedience and open homosexuality, he has continued to fight for equality. He died in New York City on August 24, 1987.

Bayard Rustin had been brought up to believe that his parents were Julia and Janifer Rustin, when in fact they were his grandparents. He discovered the truth before adolescence, that the woman he thought was his sister, Florence, was actually his mother, who had had Rustin with West Indian immigrant Archie Hopkins.

Rustin attended Wilberforce University in Ohio and Cheyney State Teachers College (now Cheney University of Pennsylvania) in Pennsylvania, both historically black schools. In 1937 he moved to New York City and studied at City College in New York. He was involved in the League of Young Communists for a short time in the 1930s, before becoming disillusioned with his activities and resigning.

In his personal philosophy, Rustin combined the pacifism of the Quaker religion, the non-violent resistance taught by Mahatma Gandhi and the socialism married to the African American labor leader A. Philip Randolph. During World War II he worked for Randolph, fighting racial discrimination in war-related hiring.

Rustin has been punished several times for his beliefs. During the war, he was jailed for two years when he refused to register for the project. When he took part in protests against the segregated public transit system in 1947, he was arrested in North Carolina and sentenced to work in a gang of chains for several weeks. In 1953 he was arrested on charges of morality for publicly engaging in homosexual activities and was sent to prison for 60 days. However, he continued to live as an openly gay man.

Rustin met young civil rights leader Dr. Martin Luther King Jr. in the 1950s and started working with King as an organizer and strategist in 1955. He taught King of Gandhi's philosophy of non-violent resistance and advised him on the tactics of civil disobedience . He assisted King in the boycott of segregated buses in Montgomery, Alabama, in 1956. In particular, Rustin was a key figure in organizing the march on Washington for Jobs and Freedom, during which King delivered his legendary speech "I Have a Dream "on August 28, 1963.

In 1965, Rustin and his mentor Randolph co-founded the A. Philip Randolph Institute, a union organization for African American union members. Rustin continued his work in the civil rights and peace movements, and was in great demand as a public speaker.

Rustin has received numerous awards and honorary degrees during his career. His writings on civil rights were published in the collection Along the Line in 1971 and in the Strategies for Freedom in 1976. He continued to talk about the importance of economic equality within the Civil Rights Movement, as well as the need for rights for gay and lesbian people. Bayard Rustin died in New York City on August 24, 1987, at the age of 75.

Rosa Louise Parks

Rosa Louise Parks (February 4, 1913 - October 24, 2005) was an African American activist engaged in the struggle for civil rights.

On December 1, 1955, Parks took a bus to return home after a day of work in Montgomery, Alabama, in the deep South. Since the only free seat was in the front of the vehicle, the one reserved for "whites" Parks went to sit there. Shortly after, some "white" passengers got on the bus and asked her arrogantly to get up and vacate the seat, as required by the segregation law of that state. Immediately she is forced to get up, but she refuses. The driver, James Blake, is called in by the police and Rosa is arrested for sitting on a place for white people.

It was the first episode of the boycott of Montgomery buses. After the arrest of Parks, a 42-year-old seamstress guilty of sitting in an empty seat on public transport, for 381 days the black people of Montgomery refused to board the buses. The boycott ended on December 21, 1956, after 382 days in duration. Meanwhile, on November 13, 1956, the United States Supreme Court declared segregation buses in Alabama unconstitutional.

Rosa Parks' simple but courageous gesture made her a symbol of the civil rights movement in the United States and around the world, an icon of the global struggle against racism and injustice.

The example of Rosa Parks teaches us that non-violent disobedience to an unjust law is right. It shows that the world can be changed even without vulgarity, without insults, without violence, without having to demonize and bring down an enemy. Even with a small but strong no.

And it makes us understand that each of us can follow the example of that woman, a simple but determined forty-two-year-old seamstress, the wife of a Montgomery barber, in the deep American South. When she published an autobiography in 1992, the woman explained the reasons for her gesture: "People always say I didn't get up because I was tired, but that's not true. I was not physically tired or more tired than usual after a day of work. I wasn't old even though some people think I was. I was 42 years old. No, the only thing I was tired of was giving in".

Mohammed Ali

Cassius Clay was one of the most important boxers in the world. Gold medal in Rome in 1960 and world heavyweight champion, Cassius Clay was born in Lousville, in the largest city in the state of Kentucky, on January 17, 1942. He approached the "noble art" at just twelve years old, noticed by a policeman from the city. Cassius Clay took a short time to show his talent: quick on his feet, quick in his movements and endowed with an extension that surprised his opponents.

Hiscareer began at the 1960 Olympics in Rome and is described encounter after encounter, sentence after sentence. Performances not only sporting, but also linguistic, word games that have made Ali an ante litteram rapper. The rise, the world title won against the bad bear Sonny Liston amid a thousand provocations and controversies, the following day the young American boxer decided to convert to the Islamic religion and change his name to Muhammad Ali.

In 1965, there was a rematch with Sonny Liston: the match went down in history for the ghost punch given by Muhammad Ali to his opponent during the first resumption of the clash and which decreed his defeat. The following years marked the domination of the American boxer who defended the world champion title 8 times.

The conversion to Islam, the proximity to Malcolm X and Martin Luther King, the refusal of the war in Vietnam. The heavyweight world champion who refuses to serve the homeland. Half America opposes it. Including strong powers. The sender of an investigative document about him makes his wrists tremble, Edgar Hoover says, he is the powerful head of the FBI.

In 1967, Muhammad Ali was sentenced to 5 years in prison for refusing to participate in the war in Vietnam, for the simple reason "They didn't call me a nigger" which also cost him the withdrawal of his boxing license.

Ali is deprived of the title, but it is also the moment when the boxer becomes an icon, a way of being, of thinking. On university campuses crowds of students flock to listen and support him. The disqualification lasts three years, the return is very hard. The Madison Teams Garden in New York, on March 8, 1971, on the occasion of the first meeting of the legendary trilogy with Joe Frazier, is a cross-section of American society. Nobody wants to miss. In the clash of the century, Ali lost in the fifteenth recovery.

The revenge between the two boxers took place on January 28, 1974. Muhammad Ali finally defeated Frazier and in October of the same year challenged Foreman for the world champion title. The match was played in Zaire, in a stadium that contained over one hundred thousand people. After a bloody fight that lasted 8 rounds, Ali managed to knock Foreman down and conquer the heavyweight crown.

When the match is played in the then Zaire, Ali is already a planetary character, a charmer of crowds, a landlord in the countless talk shows in which he participates.

The following year, the maximum champion met Frazier for the third time, this time in Manila, the Philippines: on the fifteenth round, Muhammad Ali managed to defeat the opponent. It was the boxer's last big fight from Lousville. Muhammad Ali ended his career with 56 wins in 61 games.

Only On a couple of occasions, Muhammad Ali has probably mixed some perfidy with the extraordinary boxing class. It was when he faced, and beaten, Ernie Terrell and Oscar Bonavena. Those two had called him Cassius Clay with provocative insistence, the slave name from which he did not feel represented in supporting the battles for civil rights.

First actor of a theater in which few seem to play a role congenial to them. Mohammad Ali was an icon representative of the disillusioned aspirations of black people. The decline in the ring, which materializes definitively in the defeat against the former sparring Larry Holmes, is secondary to the charisma of man.

President Carter sends him to Africa to support the boycott of the Moscow Olympics, but other presidents also compete to show up in his company. From Reagan and Clinton, the latter moved to tears when 'The Greatest', beaten by Parkinson's disease, trembles the Olympic brazier in Atlanta. When this happens, Cassius Marcellus Clay is only a memory, now there is only Muhammad Ali.

Jesse Jackson

Born on October 8, 1941, Jesse Louis Burns (Burns is the mother's surname) grew up in Greenville, South Carolina in a typical US middle-class family. His natural father, Noah Robinson, was one of the first successful African American businessmen. He did not recognize his son because he was married to another woman. Later, Jackson's mother married Charles Henry Jackson, who formally adopted little Jesse in 1957.

In 1965, Jesse Jackson joined Martin Luther King's Southern Christian Leadership Conference (SCLC) movement in Selma, Alabama. The collaboration and understanding with King confirms him as Civil Rights Leader. It has a large oratory that King decided to entrust to Jackson in 1966. He was very inspired in his actions by Martin Luther King and was in Memphis when the latter was assassinated on April 4, 1968.In the eighties, he reached great fame by imposing himself as leader of African Americans and as politician and statesman.

In June 1984, at the invitation of Fidel Castro he went to Cuba to negotiate the release of twenty-two US citizens. In 1997, Jackson flew to Kenya to meet with then-President Daniel ArapMoi as President Bill Clinton's special envoy to promote democracy through free elections.

In April 1999, during the Kosovo conflict, Jackson embarked on a trip to Belgrade to negotiate the release of three US soldiers captured on the border with the then Former Yugoslav Republic of Macedonia during a patrol action on behalf of the UN. He had a meeting with President Slobodan Milošević, who later allowed the release of the three men.

On February 15, 2003, Jackson held a rally in front of more than a million people in Hyde Park, in the heart of London, at the height of the February 15 pacifist demonstrations against the imminent invasion of Iraq by the United States and the United Kingdom.

In August 2005, Jackson reached Venezuela to meet President Hugo Chávez, and after meeting with Chávez and the Venezuelan parliament, Jackson claimed that there was no evidence that Venezuela was a threat to the United States. On his journey Jackson did not fail to meet representatives of the Afro-Venezuelan and indigenous communities.

In 1984, Jackson became the second African-American, after Shirley Chisholm, to organize a national campaign to become President of the United States, running for the Democrats. In the primaries he got 21% of the popular vote, but only 8% of the delegates.Four years later, in 1988, Jackson again offered himself as a Democratic Party primary candidate. This time, he garnered more than double the popular votes from four years earlier.

He was awarded the Colombed'Oro Peace Prize from the Disarmament Archive of Rome in 1999, with the following motivation: "The Disarmament Archive awards the international prize to Reverend Jesse Jackson, a leading exponent of the African-American community of the United States, which in the footsteps of Martin Luther King Jr., has been able to renew its commitment in defense of civil rights by integrating it with a demanding battle in favor of peace and for the development of friendship relations between all the peoples of the world.

5. HOW TO FIND OUT YOU ARE A RACIST

The test of our unconscious prejudices.

In a text of 1865, Types of Mankind, at the time considered scientific, the doctor Nott and the Egyptologist Gliddon argue, complete with illustrations, that blacks are biologically intermediate between Caucasian whites and chimpanzees. From this error, however, derives the belief that is at the basis of racism, namely that a particular group of people can be defined superior or inferior to another.

Today it is sufficient to consult internet to know that the human species cannot be subdivided into biologically distinct races, characterized by different intellectual, value or moral capacities. Racism is known to be a phenomenon as old as the world, but the fact that it can be studied on the neurobiological level is relatively recent. In collaboration with social psychologists, neuroscientists have been trying to understand how humans perceive and categorize ethnic, religious and sexual alterities for some years.These researches use brain imaging techniques to examine how our brain processes, evaluates and incorporates race and ethnicity categories into decision-making processes.

The amygdala is a nuclear complex located in the dorsomedial part of the temporal lobe of the brain that manages emotions and in particular fear. It is considered the center of integration of higher neurological processes such as emotions, also involved in the systems of emotional memory. The amygdala is therefore the archive of our emotional memory, for this it analyzes the current experience, with what has already happened in the past. When the present and past situations have a similar key element, the amygdala identifies it as an association and sometimes acts before having full confirmation.

It hastily commands us to react to a present situation according to comparisons of similar episodes, even from a long time ago, with thoughts, emotions and learned reactions fixed in response to similar events and causes repulsive reactions towards the elements considered foreign, preceded by a feeling of disgust. The amygdala can react before the cerebral cortex knows what is happening, and this is because raw emotion is unleashed independently of conscious thought, and generally before it.

The so-called IAT, Implicit Association Test, in fact, measures the reaction times to stimulus images. They are a simple and ancient way to empirically verify the unconscious share of our prejudices, reactions of disgust and aversion towards those who have a different color from ours, or another sexual orientation and so on.It is our most visceral and least human part. The defensive function of disgust fulfills the need to project our animality onto others in order to feel more human.

But the result of this defense is, paradoxically, precisely that of remaining harnessed in our most instinctive functions, fear, paranoia, control, aggression, moving away from humanity.

To let ourselves be guided by our xenophobias, homophobias, misogynies, means being dominated by primitive automatisms, ending up hating everything that, embodying our fears and the aspects of us that we reject, makes us feel insecure and threatened.

Much research helps us understand this psychological reading. For example, it shows that at the basis of many anti-homosexual attitudes there is a reaction of disgust. Those who are more prone to disgust are also more likely to disapprove of a passionate kiss between two women or two men.

And moral disapproval is likely to function as a rationalizing and reassuring defense that empowers you to voice your disgust. When moral disapproval is less viable, as in the case of racism, then other strategies can be used. It's not that I hate the Chinese, they steal our jobs "; It's not that I hate black people, they are the ones who rape our women and so on.

For a mocking coincidence of events, the murder of Gerge Floyd for most whites (Americans) takes longer to associate (IAT) images of black people with the word "good" and images of white people with the word "bad" .

And that, if we see images representing ethnic groups other than ours, brain activations take place at the amygdala level. Even more interesting is when the IAT reveals racism not so much of those who make it a political profession (the naked eye is enough here), but of those who, on the other hand, profess themselves to be anti-racist (or anti-homophobic). "I racist?"

In their deep brain or unconscious, do all whites think that blacks (or Jews, or gays) are apes? No. The "neuroscience of racism" testifies to a primitive vulnerability to the theme "belonging vs non-belonging" to what is considered one's own "group".

It is a yielding to archaic fears and feelings of inferiority. Phelps' experiments also show that tests conducted using familiar faces (African-American actors and politicians) report a decrease in amygdala activity.

And that, over time, the activation of the amygdala decreases, leaving room for a cortical elaboration of "reasoning". In short, and it is not surprising to find out, knowledge and reason are effective answers against racism.

Prejudices are within us.

We were all human beings, until religion separated us, politics divided us, the color of the skin made us enemies and money classified us.

In any case, we can say that we are absolutely against any form of discrimination but in our unconscious there is a mistrust towards those who are different. This, at least, is what Project Implicit scholars claim. An IAT test has been developed, which since the mid-nineties monitors the associations of ideas between faces and concepts. The test is divided into eight sections, each of which addresses a series of prejudices related to age, race, nationality, gender, disability, skin color, weight and sexual orientation.

In some ways it is similar to a video game. Once you have entered your data and expressed your political and religious preferences, you go to the phase of association of faces. If on the left there is written "thin" and on the right there is written "fat" and the face of a thin person appears, click on the button on the left, and vice versa with fat people.

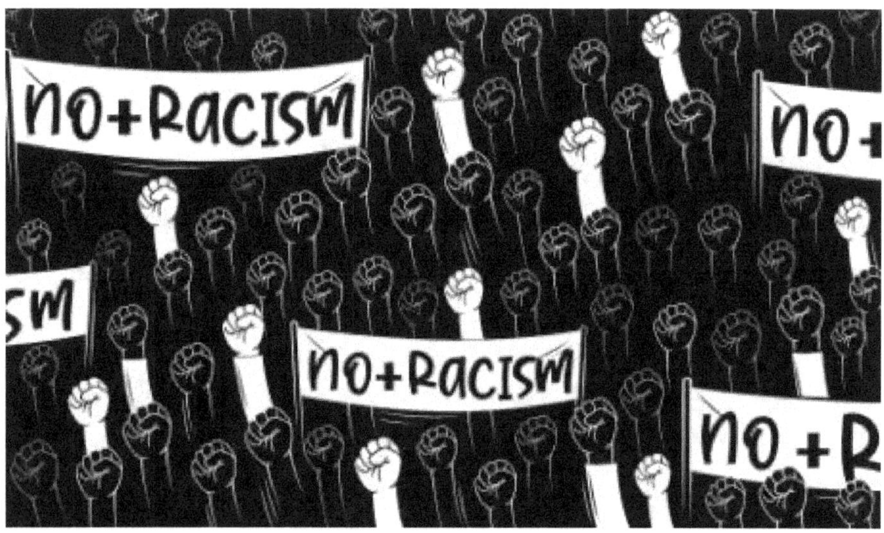

Then the concepts are associated with the same system. For example, on the left is written "good" and on the right "bad". If the word "glory" appears, the key on the left will be typed, if the right one will appear "evil".

Subsequently, in the test, the photos and concepts are interspersed, with a couple of steps that invert the position of good and evil and the division, to remain in the example of the first between thin and fat.

The result is that if you take less time to associate a positive concept with the good after you have just associated a thin face, you will have a preference for thin people. And vice versa. If it sounds too complicated, just go to the Harvard University website and you can try the test.

A lot is being said about this experiment in the United States, where after the various events that have followed, including tragic ones, tensions and accusations of police officers and judges of having racial prejudices have multiplied. In the interpretation that of the test, there is precisely the need to be aware of the existence of even unconscious prejudices that could concern those who are required to judge or maintain public order.

Unfortunately, tests have in fact confirmed that "implicit bias", a mechanism by which our mind implicitly leads us to prefer or have a negative preconception, towards a group of people with a common trait, which can be their religion, ethnicity, are still very present.

One of the most curious aspects of the research is that, although the prejudices are greater towards people of different ethnic backgrounds, there are also intra-group prejudices. So while white Americans generally have implicit prejudices against other ethnic groups, even those belonging to minorities may have prejudices against their group.

This implies that the situation could improve. The approach to reduce prejudices even at a deep level is that which involves contact with people who challenge stereotypes or with individuals and groups with whom we have unconscious prejudices. The earlier you start, the better.

Implicit Association Test (IAT)

In short, making a serious self-analysis is a very valid method to measure the racist rate that lodges at various levels within each of us. Just do a simple online search to undergo the Implicit Association Test (IAT). It is a very reliable psychological test that describes racists and the unconscious.

Obviously, the results of the IAT should not be confused with the ideas that everyone has about the world. There is a heated debate in the scientific world on the weight to be given to this experiment, and on how to interpret the results.

It is a fairly accepted idea that a very high implicit bias does not necessarily lead to discriminatory behavior. It has been discovered that the correlation between implicit bias and discriminatory behavior is weaker than previously thought, and that there is very little evidence that changes in implicit bias have anything to do with changes in a person's behavior.

If even in the scientific world we wonder about the actual interpretation to be given to the results of the IAT, nobody doubts that it is a precious parameter to understand something more about how our unconscious discriminatory schemes work.

People are often shocked by the results obtained by the IAT, because many times they think they are not racist. By doing this test, however, they have the opportunity to verify and examine their prejudice and the fact of obtaining unflattering results for many is a motivation to commit and try to change their attitudes.

Racists without knowing it: The Passing

Passing is the ability to conceal one's racial identity to take on a new one. It is a thorny subject in America, deeply linked to racism against blacks, racial segregation and the attempt to choose how to be considered.

The first example of passing in America dates back to the very first migratory wave of Indians. Essentially men who arrived in the late nineteenth century to sell hand-embroidered fabrics, to whites with the mania of the Orient. They often ended up marrying white, black or Hispanic women and giving birth to new American families.

The dualism typical of the way of looking at races in America caused much confusion among whites on how to classify Indians and their descendants. They were not black, but certainly not white. They lent themselves more to being welcomed among whites, marked as exotic and flattered for their oriental merchandise. Some black men discovered that wearing turbans and adopting Muslim names allowed them to cross the border between Negro and Hindu, going from a disparaged diversity to an exotic one. With black skin that became socially acceptable when it had previously been inadmissible, it didn't mean much, but it did increase the chances of social survival for some.

However, passing depends not only on the appearance you have, but also on the context and people you surround yourself with. Due to their dark complexion, Indians were often welcome in Hispanic and African American neighborhoods and communities. At the time of getting married, many chose black and Hispanic women. The census officer was confused about what a Hindu was and marked the couple and their offspring as belonging to his wife's ethnic group. Things would change a few years later with the Expatriation Act of 1907, with which women took citizenship of husbands regardless of residence.

The Story of an Indian Woman.

I turned black when I was nine years old when I came to France and met whites. You become black with the eyes of others. Lilian Thuram states in his book "My black stars". A young American, Jaya Saxena, of Indian origins, talks about racism, cultural stereotypes and the thin border line between who we are and how others see us.

Racism is in the eye of the beholder and the context allows people to make assumptions and also determines whether they play in favor of the person concerned or not. Although people have asked me all my life "what" I am, I never know the answer to this question until someone else gives it to me. My father was a doctor, with fairer skin than mine. In the family it is said that they had often mistaken him for a Jew.

For whites, I am white like them until proven otherwise, and once the truth is revealed, they always assure me with enthusiasm that I can still go for one of them. I heard about my physical expectation that on a winter's day in low light I could even be mistaken for a Frenchwoman.

For black people, it is usually evident that there is something non-white about me. The shape of the eyes or the black hair or something else. But even for black people I represent an ethnic unknown sort, and usually those who watch me tend to mistake me for what I hope I am.

Like many wealthy university colleagues, after graduation I spent a few months traveling alone to unknown places. I was convincing myself to give a purpose in life. In a hostel, an Israeli boy approached me and started trying to speak with me in Hebrew, as I sensed by his expression and the gestures he made with his hands. So I said in English, "Sorry, I don't speak Hebrew." He was stunned: "But if you're Jewish!" He exclaimed, a conclusion he had jumped on his own. It happened everywhere. In New Zealand they were convinced that I had Maori blood. In Chile they thought I was a local who carried tourists around. In the Greek neighborhood where I live, they often mistake me for a second generation snob who has never learned Greek. And every time someone guesses wrong, I'm the one who apologizes.

There is no need for people to know that I am Indian. It has nothing to do with my face or skin, with my religion or my daily habits. I could choose an English name and simply become another white girl who loves Indian food and bracelets.

This of course would mean denying my family and my cultural heritage and all those invisible little things that make me Indian, and I would never do such a thing. But being able to reveal your racial identity instead of being identified right away has an advantage. You become a nice surprise, fascinating and fantastic for people who feel normal, and therefore boring.

Once, in a bar, I introduced myself to a woman I was playing pool with. After the inevitable question about my name followed by the usual answer, the woman screamed with joy. "India is so beautiful," she insisted, so enchanting and full of colors and many other typical things. She asked me what I thought of The Millionaire even though I never said I saw it. It was all very annoying, but at least I was the different "exotic" and not the one despised.

Usually this thing about having to reveal one's identity is the consequence of an error made by someone else, and is accompanied by the embarrassment of informing the interlocutor of being wrong. And also, in a way, to be wrong. Our face, our ways, the color of our skin have hidden the truth giving others the wrong impression, and it is as if we had embarrassed them. Too much education sometimes has the effect of reversing responsibilities up to this point.

When I declare who I am, what I am, whether it's in a tweet or an essay or in a conversation, I do it because nobody blames me for a half-truth. To never confirm the wrong assumptions of the women who frequent the parks, I learned to immediately declare my racial identity, before someone has the opportunity to ask me questions, to summarize four hundred years of my family history so that no one is wrong. So that I'm not wrong.

With the intent to rekindle the fear of black people, President Trump has brought these thoughts back to the center of my life. I don't run the risk of a stranger drawing a swastika on my door.

Many biased people who work in the tertiary sector may simply think that I owe my name to two hippie parents. My husband, who is Jewish, has received many more racial insults on the Internet than I have. Unless I manifest it, nobody can see the fear I have for my father, who does not yet have citizenship, or my grandmother, who never wears western clothes.

I have three different racial identities: white, Indian and multiracial. In me there is not one that prevails over the others. They are all complete and part of me in the same way. I feel white when people accuse whites of racism and demand that they change their attitude. I feel Indian who prompts them to make their voices heard in places where they hold power. I feel like a mixed race person who reminds everyone that cultural superstructures, apparently so solid, collapse at the slightest closer examination.

CONCLUSION

The book suggests some practical tips to try, if not to solve the problem of racism at least to stem it. It is a very effective contribution because it fully illustrates the situation that has arisen in the USA, from a social, economic and political point of view. The reason is very simple, if you know a topic, it is much easier to understand it and if it is appropriate to intervene to correct it. The first step is to take action on yourself.

Racism is difficult to eradicate, like any other bad habit. There will probably never be any prejudice and it may be necessary to work for a long time to eradicate this social offense. Almost all people, even if they do not blatantly endorse racism, have some kind of prejudice towards a group of people, of which they are not even aware. For this reason, defeating racism becomes increasingly difficult.

Sometimes this aversion gives rise to anger and personal and social violence. However, overcoming the racist mentality is possible even if it requires a long path to follow, on a personal and collective level. Just follow some tips to intervene first of all on yourself and then work on others. Racism is won if we change things starting from ourselves and from the community we live in.

We must intervene whenever we witness an episode of racism. It is necessary to support and attend events dedicated to the different cultures in the world and to spend for the approval and application of anti-discrimination laws. Participating in the debate and intervening with personal anti-racist beliefs is very important to produce results conducive to integration. It is a very delicate topic, because there is the risk of losing some friends and family members, who are not very sensitive to anti-racist problems, who may not appreciate the commitment to overcome this prejudice.

For the same reason, some racist attitude is assumed, for sheer consistency, it is desirable to apologize and try to understand why you have fallen into error, instead of making false reasons.

We must ensure that history does not repeat itself again and that in the future Human Rights begin to assert themselves in every single person, in the neighborhood where you live, in the school you attend, and in every factory, farm or office in the world.

COMPULSIVE EATING

How to overcome binge-eating-disorders and re-program your brain to stop being obsessed by hunger. A guide to develop self-confidence by maintaining a mindful and healthy relationship with food.

ADELE ADANI

"There are people in the world so hungry, that God cannot appear to them except in the form of bread."

Mahatma Gandhi.

INTRODUCTION

Compulsive behaviors can be defined as repeated attitudes, despite being inadequate in certain situations. People often recognize that their behavior is harmful, but they feel emotionally compelled to implement it. Compulsion, in general, is linked to obsessive-compulsive disorder, in the non-control of the impulses of substance abuse.

However compulsive behavior is a *modus operandi* not only of substance abuse from addictions, but also of eating disorders, such as the Binge Eating Disorder.

This pathology linked to food is characterized by an immoderate and uncontrollable need to overeat. The control of this behavior is very difficult, despite the attempts undertaken.

The current models to counter the Binge Eating Disorder focus attention on three elements in particular:

1) uncontrolled feeding as a habit;

2) nutrition as a dysfunctional strategy to deal with a negative emotional state;

3) uncontrolled nutrition despite adverse consequences.

Compulsive feeding is characterized by brain dysfunctions in the areas dedicated to learning by reward. The reward system is a group of neural structures responsible for motivation, associative learning and positive emotions, in particular, those that involve pleasure such as, joy, euphoria and ecstasy.

The reward is the motivational property of a stimulus that induces appetitive behavior, also known as consumption behavior, which flows into the Binge Eating Disorder. Understanding how and why this disturbing complex develops is very difficult.

It is good to be wary of those who claim to know what the causes of these ailments are. The reasons are many and probably different from person to person. Although research is becoming increasingly interested in this topic, numerous efforts are still needed to hinder compulsive eating behavior.

Our work aims to improve the prospects of prevention and treatment in a preventive perspective, probing the emotional processes in charge of controlling feelings.

Feelings and emotions live with us, yet many times we pay little attention to our inner experience. We do not see our emotional world as a wealth, a potential. We are more inclined to enhance rational thinking, leaving aside the emotional experience.

In the era in which we find ourselves living, characterized by the desire to posses more, everything immediately in real time, the time for self-reflection is every time less. We live, in fact, in an accelerated world in which everyone is always in a hurry. To understand what is really important it is necessary to stop, re-evaluate ourselves and revisit the emotions experienced. Our experiences accompany us and silently challenge us, call us back, guide us. So it is important to consider emotional dynamisms to better penetrate emotions and evaluate how much they can help us embark on a new lifestyle.

This work is proposed as an attempt to re-evaluate this re-marriage that we have available. The book is divided into six chapters and tries to give useful information for those who, taken by their health problems, seem to ignore every other sphere of humanity and pay attention to feelings and emotions. They therefore grow as emotionally illiterate. They selfishly focus on the relationship of the senses, touch, smell, and of course, above all the taste, which obviously deals with food.

All this must be educated, it must be exercised, it must be formed through constancy and listening to oneself in order to open up to the other. The book will be a training journey to glimpse how, by listening to wisely evaluated advice and indications, it is possible to reach the goal of embarking on a path of authentic socio-affective integration. A part of the book will go into the various ways of countering the Binge Eating Disorder one of the most common ailments in the modern population.

It is a story of the difficult struggle to get out of the disease that affects people and involves their families. Obviously, for a scientific and professional approach to the Binge Eating Disorder, the support of a team of experts is the only solution for the administration of appropriate treatments and therapies to be followed, to effectively tackle the various pathologies. A widely documented reconstruction of all the stages of this long obstacle course has been made, in which food, the body and emotions are the fundamental tools for the rebirth of a new life.

The message is to remember that it is always possible to transform our weak points into an opportunity for growth and gift. Believing that situations of fatigue, anguish, sadness, pain are always in us and give meaning to our life. The realization of the person consisting in continually reaching more, integrated with what he already has, allows you to take a step forward in your existential journey.

1. WE ARE WHAT WE EAT

Philosophy and Food

Eating is universal and the universal, you know, pleases philosophy. However at the same time it has to do with the body, as well as sexuality. Eating goes beyond the biological question and opens up to the dimension of meaning.

Philosophy has always dealt with food, understood both as the primary need of the body and as a metaphor for what nourishes the human. Through the food act, we become what we eat.

The philosophical approach has allowed us to interpret food through a subjective, relational and natural point of view.

Nourishment stimulates our subjective sphere, reassures us and brings us back to the metaphor of the original contact, the maternal one. The analysis of subjectivity within the relationship with food reveals an inevitable relationship with the other. The socio-relational path starts from the maternal body up to the food community to which the individual feels he belongs and which he contributes to determining.

By taking food we assimilate the world is also the comparison with the animal, with whom we share the need for nourishment and consequently the act of eating. Through the alimentary act, we become what we eat. This is a comparison that depresses humans to the bestial condition, flattening them at the level of simple matter. As in other areas, also in relation to food, man is constantly engaged in developing strategies that could definitively indicate a detachment from the animal world.

Medieval thought judges excess food as lust, particularly forms of intemperance of the senses. They are both transgressions of the flesh, respectively, inherent in excess in the food and sexual spheres.

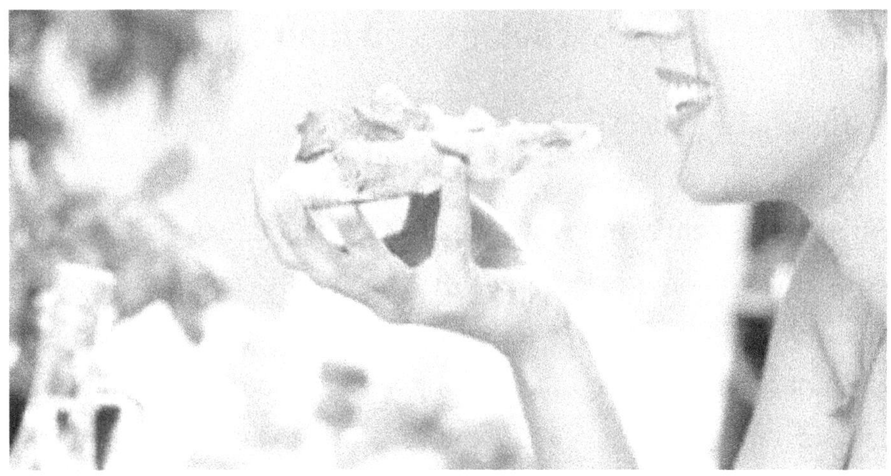

The act of eating is necessarily connected to pleasure. It is difficult to distinguish what is required from necessity and pleasure. Given the physiological need for nourishment, we should be able to discern between need and desire. In the act of eating, we satisfy two types of appetite, the natural appetite, to which belong the primary sensations of hunger and thirst, which refers to need. At the same time, we satisfy the sensory appetite, which presides over the desire for food and tastes.

If we want, this classification allows us to identify the fate of the insatiable from those of the voracious, which sometimes coincides with those affected by the binge eating disorder.

The first has to do with the qualitative refinement of the senses, it does not satisfy itself for the materiality of the food, but for the unbridled exaltation of the sensations of the palate. The second has to do not only with the satisfaction of the physiological need but with the excessive quantity of hunger, therefore, the insatiability of the natural appetite.

Psychology and food

Those affected by binge eating seem to ignore every other sphere of humanity, paying limited attention to the feelings and emotions. Leave out your inner experience, your emotional world. They therefore grow as emotionally illiterate, unrelated to themselves and to what happens inside them, wrapped in a storm of emotions from which they are increasingly dominated and less and less able to learn. Thus we lose contact with that part of us without which it is difficult to lead a peaceful life. He selfishly focuses on the relationship of the senses, the touch, the sense of smell and, of course, above all the taste, which relate it to food. Consequently, the act of eating can be automatic and at the same time full of irreversible consequences, which escape the control and moderation of reason.

The separation between body and reason that has marked philosophy since its inception has meant that philosophy has given only marginal importance to food.

Although once those who ate excessively were opposed, in the eyes of modern sensibility, they no longer seem to be attributable to such a serious lack. Gluttony, from capital transgression, a moral error worthy of eternal punishment has become, for men of the beginning of the third millennium, a venial infringement of the aesthetic order.

To the ethical imperatives of the societies of hunger and shortage, the modern civilization of consumption has replaced the prescriptions, sometimes just as iron and binding for the needs of fashion and the public to appear, of dietetics. They therefore grow as emotionally illiterate, extraneous to themselves and to what happens inside them, wrapped in a storm of emotions from which they are increasingly dominated and less and less able to learn. In the era in which we find ourselves living, characterized by the tendency to want everything immediately in real time, little time is reserved for reflection on oneself. We live, in fact, in an accelerated world in which everyone is always in a hurry, while to understand what is really important it is necessary to stop, re-evaluate, understand with the emotions experienced. Our experiences accompany us, silently challenge us, call us back, guide us. So the intelligence of emotions remains an educational challenge for everyone. Indeed, emotion is not only what happens to us, but above all it is what moves us. So it is important to consider emotional dynamisms. We must not only understand emotions, but evaluate how much these emotions can help us understand.

The message is to remember that it is always possible to transform our weak points into an opportunity for growth and gift, to believe that in situations of fatigue, anguish, sadness pain there is a sense for one's existence, because the realization of the person consists in reaching continuously what more, integrated with what it already has, allows you to take a step forward in our existential journey.

The Consumer Society

In today's obese society there is a perverse combination between the physical feeling of satisfaction and fullness on the one hand and the idea of obeying the norms of insatiable consumption on the other.

To the society of overproduction, much more than bodies that work, they are interested in the bodies that consume. The spirit of capitalism stimulates, the tendency to insatiability and awakens different forms of desire for accumulation.

Everything is mobilized to awaken an ever new hunger, not only for food. An important component of our day is the intake of the products of the media diet. We start from the poorest, consisting only of television and we get to the slightly more moderate one based on TV, radio and newspapers up to the diet rich in new technologies.

Another type of hunger is involved in this area, metaphorically fueled by the connection network, hunger for devices to be consumed, which the appropriate sales centers present, by virtue of shrewd marketing strategies. The sales techniques flatter and pamper the customer, making him feel unique and loved, and present in design packages, true design masterpieces. Therefore both food and electronic gadgets appear to some to be the only thing that can take care of them. For the physiological appetite, the mechanisms are identical. Satisfaction is found in the sweet-soft fat diet, easy and cheap, where the overweight person obediently bends to the ideal of the insatiable consumer who feeds on low-cost foods rich in calories, sugars and fats, salt and yeast.

The mass consumption industry contributes to the spread of food illiteracy and the inability to cook good food, with style and competence, without falling into the trap of the rhetoric of the grandmother's kitchen.

Sedentary lifestyle

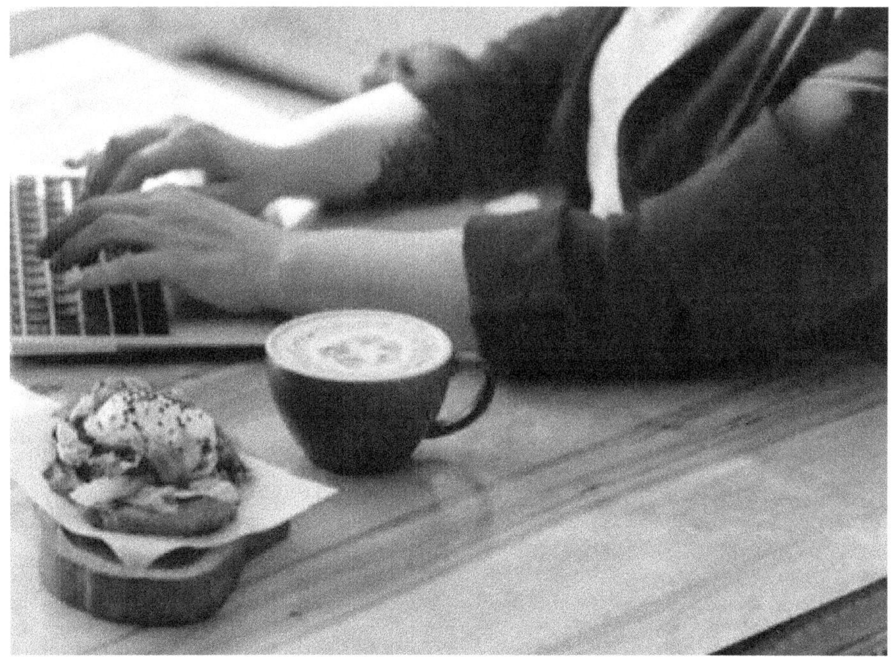

Sedentary lifestyle and poor nutrition contribute significantly to the increase in obesity. The opportunities for physical activity have been reduced by the introduction of technological instruments such as elevators, cars and remote controls. We spend more time on sedentary activities, such as using the computer, watching television and playing video games. In addition, the types of work have become more sedentary. Work in the office or at the desk has replaced manual work. Those who lead a sedentary lifestyle need fewer calories than more active people and therefore require a diet with a lower calorie intake. If the latter is not reduced, weight is gained.

Stereotypes society

It is a new society today, a 2.0 society, of self-care and self-diagnosis. A society in which stereotypes and prejudices are the masters, especially with regards to external beauty. Today, in fact, a body is defined as beautiful only when it is able to wear tight sizes and trendy clothes.

All this has consequences. To look beautiful, you need to be online and follow diets, most often found on websites or by famous people who promote their healthy diet. Strange diets, accompanied by supplements and pseudo-drugs that guarantee excellent results in a short time. Diets that through a few steps, can be found and available to everyone, without being calibrated on the person, without particular medical visits and without being prescribed by specialists in the sector.

Contentment and satisfaction for one's body have always been topics treated and considered almost an obsession. In the beginning, this was mainly visible in the female. Today, however, it seems that the male world has adopted these nuances, but in a different way. The lack of fulfillment for males focuses on a lack or lack of muscles or poorly defined physicality. In women it focuses on thinness or elimination of fat mass. In fact, for these and other reasons, eating disorders such as Bulimia, Anorexia, Vomiting and Binge Eating mainly affect the female population, even if there are significant exceptions.

Eating disorders are described as pathologies characterized by alterations in eating habits and by excessive concern about one's image, in particular weight and body shapes.

Social Reactions

Social reactions to obese people are often negative. The obese arouses anger. A social weight appears, surrounded by depressing prejudices like a greedy, lazy being, without self-control. Often people avoid sitting nearby on public transport. Comedians don't feel the need to hold back in their jokes. We imagine that in the near future the obese will be able to consider themselves subject to discrimination and believe they are stalking victims. And that the word fat will be considered politically incorrect.

Even in past, a limited number of obese did not represent a social problem, nor require health policy interventions. Indeed, people in the flesh enjoyed a particular social prestige and their body mass inspired confidence, as well as representing, in some eras, an ideal of beauty.

Since then, psychology has taken matters into its own hands. Together with the natural and anthropometric sciences, which give normality increasingly exact weights, shapes and volumes. And at the same time the language also creates neologisms to define in an ever more detailed way those intermediate states between fat and thin that previously had no name. Diminutive and augmentative, such as plump, rotund, fleshed, corpulent, plump, fat, which are in fact personal words, calibrating judgments.

These over sizes are the pariahs of the global village. First, I took my throat from the planetary junk food market, of which they are the insatiable financiers. And then stigmatized by a system that points to public condemnation as compulsive omnivores, unproductive parasites, unwilling subjects, time bombs for the health system, unsustainable overweight for welfare. How to say humiliated and obese. And also punished.

So much so that they earn on average eighteen percent less than normal weight. This is shown, figures in hand, by a recent Swedish research. However, obesity is not a disease that strikes at random regardless of eating habits and lifestyle.

Food Ignorance

In industrialized countries, nutrition consists of foods that contain many calories in a relatively small amount. Most of these foods contain a higher amount of refined carbohydrates and fats, and a lower amount of fiber.

Ready-made foods, such as high-calorie snacks available at vending machines and fast-food restaurants, contribute to the increase in obesity. High-calorie drinks, including sodas, juices, many coffee-based drinks and alcohol, also contribute significantly.

Larger portions served in restaurants and prepackaged food and drinks encourage you to consume too much food. In addition, the foods served in restaurants and packaged ones often have high-calorie preparations, therefore, it is possible that you consume a large amount of calories without realizing it.

Food hurts when we ingest too much and too often, and then because a large part of the food we ingest is bad, not genuine, adulterated, sophisticated. A person who consciously feeds on good food will not tend to obesity. By good food we mean moderate portions, homemade preparations starting from simple and poorly treated ingredients, eating at least once a day, at regular times sitting at a table and possibly in company.

Consuming good food is avoiding buying in the supermarket and offering children as calming packs of bottles of sweet and carbonated drinks, preserved and sugary fruit juices, elaborate packaged products such as chips, snacks and sweets.

Critical Consumption of Food

Across the western world, but not only, the growth in the percentage of obese people is increasingly dramatic. The consequence of their condition is to become seriously ill. If the main culprits of overweight have been identified for some time in Junk food and carbonated drinks, a serious information campaign to avert the danger has not yet been started.

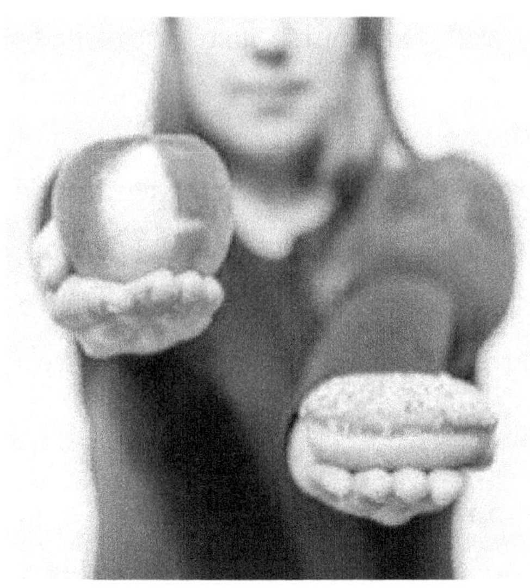

Many people still have not understood how genuine food choices can represent the only real protection against heart attacks, hypertension, stroke, diabetes and therefore be a guarantee of health and longevity. If the institutions provided information on the link between the so-called wellness diseases, hypertension, diabetes, cardiovascular problems and a diet rich in meat and dairy products, a gradual change in lifestyle and the burden of health costs would be induced. The public would shrink.

It would be appropriate to introduce the teaching of notions of nutrition and healthy and genuine gastronomy in the didactic programs. However, the resistance to such a radical change is still very strong, both from public opinion and from institutions, thanks to the very powerful industrial food lobbies,

The truth is that we are still tied to the myth of the flesh, to the idea that it is indispensable. Concepts and prejudices that are as entrenched as they are wrong. We eat meat thinking that it is the basis of nourishment. A steak provides protein and iron, but in equal if not less quantities than legumes. In addition it contains cholesterol and saturated fats, totally absent from the vegetable option.

Then, it is appropriate to reiterate that too often people forget that today we eat chickens built in the laboratory, modified in DNA. Their meats are 3 times fatter than those of old chickens and imbued with toxic substances deriving from antibiotics and hormones administered to chickens in large quantities and irresponsibly. Public canteens should provide for the introduction of an option as an alternative to dishes containing animal products or ingredients.

However, most doctors still claim the usefulness of feeding on meat. When they prescribe a diet they do not eliminate it but they prescribe lean meat, without sauces, without fats. While generally when eating meat, for the sake of the taste of the palate, we eat very seasoned meat, many sausages, chops. Nobody eats unseasoned chicken. Only those who are on a diet, in fact. But when it comes to eating meat, we are not talking about uncooked chicken, but more tasty and fatty meat. However, given the proven huge environmental impact of meat, the problem will have to be addressed. It is not possible to go ahead and take resources from the planet just to satisfy the palate.

Consequently, it is appropriate for the medical world, in a more scientific and objective way, to affirm that cereals, legumes, vegetables and fruit are able to provide the necessary for our organism a balanced nutritional intake.

Keep an eye on the food we eat, be careful, this seems to be the warning to follow. It is important to also keep in mind our environmental footprint, i.e. the production of greenhouse gases and the indiscriminate and increasingly unsustainable withdrawal of resources water, land, from the planet, by the meat industry. People need to be offered the diets they need to lead healthy lives, to fight obesity and being overweight, especially in countries that import most of their food. Excessive consumption of highly processed and high salt, sodium, sugars and trans fats imported foods is the main trigger of this situation. Estimates indicate that today 2.6 billion people are overweight and that the prevalence of obesity in the world population increased from 11.7 percent in 2012 to 13.2 percent in 2019.

If we don't take urgent action to stop the growth in obesity rates, we will soon have more obese people than undernourished in the world. There are several factors that favor this global obesity pandemic, and unhealthy diets are among the most significant.

First of all, there is the increased availability and ease of access to highly energetic foods rich in fats, sugars and salt, whose sales have been favored by intense advertising and marketing campaigns.

Fast-food and junk food are the best examples of this. This type of food is cheaper and easier to access than fresh food, especially for the poorest in urban areas. When resources for food start to run low, people choose cheaper foods, often high in calories but low in nutrients.

The Front of Food

Therefore on the food front there is a battle between itself and the world, between nature and culture. The struggle between control and impulsivity, between health and disease, is fought. On the food front, there are borders, limits and possibilities, between subjectivity and social relationship. In this context, many individual strategies compensating for our contradictions find space and many of the anxieties that are being generated are channeled.

The food front is also an extreme defense. In a world where you can no longer control anything, where you have lost all certainty and the possibility of self-determination, it is easy to fall into the trap of hyper-control. Through diet, it may happen that an attempt is made to restore a sort of existential balance that one feels he has lost.

Food restriction, brought to its extreme consequences, can lead to anorexia. Conversely, food overabundance, brought to its extreme consequences can lead to bulimia, obesity and binge-eating-disorder.

Critical food consumption is capable of regaining a balancing dimension, understood as a critical exercise on controlling the quality and quantity of food, which one feels to have lost.

The risk is that the battle to achieve proper nutrition produces an ever wider barrier between the self and the world. It is possible to restore a right relationship with food, in a world that produces overabundance but also food risk. The answer to this question needs a multidisciplinary perspective that sees the contribution of sociologists, psychologists, psychiatrists, anthropologists and experts in the field.

However, scientific research has taken many steps in recent years and models have been created to understand which pathways lead to disease and which factors increase the risk of getting sick.

2. EATING BEHAVIOR DISORDERS

Eating disorders are pathologies characterized by an alteration of eating habits and by an excessive concern for weight and body shapes.

They affect all people of all ages. They arise mainly during adolescence, especially female, with regard to certain pathologies such as anorexia and bulimia.

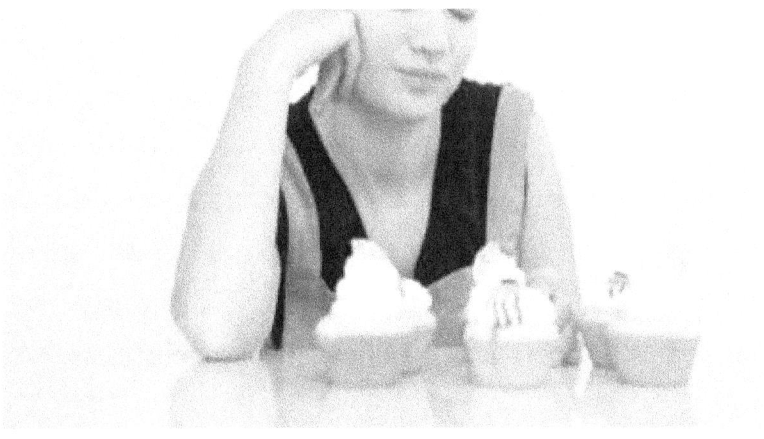

The typical behaviors of an eating disorder are revealed with the decrease in food intake, with fasting and bulimic crises. A significant amount of food is ingested in a short period of time, vomiting, the use of anorectic agents, laxatives are used and intense physical activity is used, in order to control weight.

Some people may resort to one or more of these behaviors, but this does not necessarily mean that they suffer from an eating disorder. There are in fact very specific diagnostic criteria that clarify what is to be understood as pathological.

Suffering from an eating disorder upsets a person's life and limits his or her relationship, work and social skills. For the person suffering from an eating disorder everything revolves around food and the fear of gaining weight. Things that once seemed trivial now become difficult and cause for anxiety.

Thoughts about food often haunt the person even when he is not at the table, for example at school or at work. Completing a task can become very difficult because in the head there seems to be room only for thoughts on what to eat, on the fear of gaining weight or having a bulimic crisis.

Only a small percentage of people suffering from an eating disorder ask for help. Sometimes people get complimented during their initial weight loss and this can reinforce the feeling of doing the right thing. On the other hand, when things start to worry, for the exaggerate weight loss or otherwise, it involves an important change in the person. This could start a panic crisis.

Generally, it is the family members who, first of all, alarmed by excessive weight loss, realize that something is wrong. Even for them, however, it is not easy to interfere, especially when the daughter or son does not yet have any awareness of the problem.

Not recognizing that you have a problem or using the symptoms of an eating disorder to try to solve your difficulties can have important consequences on requesting treatment.

An almost always present feature in those suffering from an eating disorder is the alteration of the body image which can become a real disorder. The perception that the person has of his own appearance or the way in which the idea of his body and forms was formed in his mind, seem to influence his life more than his real image.

Often the eating disorder is associated with other psychiatric diseases, in particular depression, but also anxiety disorders, alcohol or substance abuse, obsessive-compulsive disorder and personality disorders. Self-attacking behaviors may be present, such as self-injurious acts, such as scratching or cutting oneself up to obtain small injuries, burning parts of the body, and suicide attempts. This type of ailments occupy a very particular area in the field of psychiatry, since in addition to affecting the mind and therefore causing intense mental suffering, they also involve the body with sometimes very serious physical complications.

The main eating disorders are anorexia, bulimia, obesity and binge-eating-disorder, BED.

Anorexia

The term anorexia derives from the Greek "anorexia" and literally means lack of appetite. However, this is not an entirely appropriate definition, as the central node of anorexia is not the fact of not feeling hungry but a pathological desire to be thin.

Anorexia consists in the loss or reduction of appetite. The anorexic person despite being slim and having a weight lower than the values considered normal continues not to accept his body always seeing himself as fat.

Poor nutrition or even the resulting fasting can cause serious damage to the endocrine system leading to the absence of menstruation in women with serious consequences for fertility or increasing the risk of heart disease and osteoporosis. It mainly affects the female sex in the adolescent bracket.

For those who drop below 40 kg, they risk death from heart complications. Obviously, anorexia should not be seen only as an aesthetic dislike but must be considered an internal malaise. People suffering from anorexia nervosa are therefore underweight due to a strong decrease in food intake.

Those suffering from Anorexia often do not realize their thinness, rather they are terrified of the idea of gaining weight and becoming fat. They try to have a very strict discipline on the control of food and one's weight. People with Anorexia also give excessive weight and body shapes to assess themselves, as if their self-esteem depended on being thin and being able to control their diet.

Another feature of Anorexia in women is amenorrhea, that is, the lack of the menstrual cycle for at least three consecutive months due to weight loss and food restriction. Even when the person regains weight in some cases it takes some time before the menstrual cycle returns to being regular.

Often the disease can begin gradually and sneakily. For example, a girl can start eating a little less for different reasons.

She may lose a few extra pounds, for general digestive problems, physical ailments or surgery. It is common for the onset of the disorder to be preceded by stressful events or by important changes in life or residence, breakdown of a romantic relationship or school difficulties.

There are two different forms of anorexia, one defined as "restrictive" in which weight loss and control are due to fasting, food restriction and sometimes excessive physical activity.

Other defined compensation behaviors are characterized by the presence of bulimic crisis, together with fasting, and have the purpose of decreasing body weight. Self-induced vomiting can come through the use of improper use of diuretics or laxatives.

These two forms also differ from a psychological point of view. The restrictive form is often characterized by rigidity, obstinacy, perfectionism and obsessive-compulsive spectrum disorders and has a more favorable prognosis. The bulimic-purgative form is often accompanied by intense psychic discomfort, depression and impulsive behavior.

Bulimia

Bulimia, literally "ox hunger", is characterized by the presence of bulimic or binge crises, followed by compensatory behaviors aimed at hindering weight gain.

To reach a diagnosis of Bulimia Nervosa all the following diagnostic criteria, DSM 5 Diagnostic and Statistical Manual of Mental Disorders, must be present.

You eat more food in a certain period of time than most people would eat at the same time. You have the feeling that you are unable to stop eating or to control what and how much you are eating, followed by binge eating compensatory behaviors. Recurrent and inappropriate compensatory behaviors are used to prevent weight gain, such as self-induced vomiting, abuse of laxatives, diuretics or other drugs, fasting or excessive physical activity. Self-esteem levels are unduly influenced by the shape and weight of the body.

Bulimia Nervosa

Some people think they are bulimic because they think they overeat. In reality, the bulimic crisis, whose fundamental characteristic is Bulimia Nervosa, has very specific criteria. Thinking of exaggerating with a few more slices of dessert or ice cream certainly does not represent a real bulimic crisis.

A binge falls within the diagnostic criteria for Bulimia, when the person eats an objectively abundant amount of food in a given period of time, 1-2 hours, having the feeling of losing control and not being able to stop.

Usually the binges are made with foods considered prohibited such as sweets, carbohydrates and fats, foods that outside of binges, people with Bulimia try to eliminate from their diet. Bulimic crises must occur at least twice a week.

There are two subtypes of bulimia, the purgative and the non-purgative one. The purgative form is characterized by the presence of elimination conduits such as self-induced vomiting, by the improper use of diuretics, laxatives or enemas. Vomiting can be induced through mechanical stimulation of the throat or through the ingestion of fluids or compression of the stomach.

In the non-purgative form, the compensation methods are fasting or excessive exercise, but vomiting or other forms of purgative compensation are not regularly present. All compensatory behaviors, in any form, interfere and significantly condition the lives of people suffering from this disorder.

People with Bulimia Nervosa usually have a normal weight, although in some cases they may be overweight. A very important factor in the onset of Bulimia Nervosa is diet.

Often those who suffer from Bulimia outside of binges try to follow a very restricted diet, starting an alternating cycle of diet and bulimic crisis that consolidates and maintains the disorder itself. In some cases, bulimic crises, a low-calorie diet, follow a set of unpleasant sensations and emotions such as loneliness, boredom, anger. These are all tensions that the person manages with difficulty.

Psychological Characteristics

Often the onset of Bulimia occurs following a low-calorie diet or following a stressful event or a real emotional trauma. If at first the bulimic crisis can be occasional or occasional over time it becomes a compulsion that is difficult to escape.

In Bulimia Nervosa, attention and dissatisfaction with one's body and physical aspect can assume absolute importance. Self-esteem is strongly linked to the body and any physical modification can be experienced as a frustration and as a loss of control over one's body.

The emotional consequences of a binge can be different. In some cases, people report experiencing temporary relief and a sense of pleasure. As in most of the eating disorders in which bulimic crises are found, usually these erroneously positive effects are soon replaced by a deep anguish for the possibility of gaining weight and because you have not managed to control yourself. Compensation methods, especially vomiting, can give the temporary sensation of alleviating anxiety but afterwards a sense of emptiness may appear which in turn can trigger a new binge.

An almost always present feeling is that of shame and guilt. And this is why the disease is often hidden from family and friends for as long as possible and in many cases the request for help is made after a long time after the trouble has started.

Bulimia Nervosa not only changes eating habits, but also other important areas of the person's life. It can happen to give up the social situations that involve being at the table with others, or to become anxious and irritable and make relationships with others very difficult and tense.

Bulimia Nervosa is often associated with other mental disorders such as depression, such as substance abuse, anxiety disorders, social phobia, obsessive compulsive disorder, panic disorder and personality disorders. It is not uncommon for self-aggressive behavior such as suicide attempts or self-harming acts to occur.

Psychologically affected people with bulimia nervosa exhibit certain characteristics such as perfectionism. Often it is expressed in the imposition of very high levels of expectation both in daily life and in the objectives related to nutrition. Anything that deviates from absolute success is considered a failure and can weaken a very low and vulnerable self-esteem in most of the times.

The "all or nothing" thought is expressed with the tendency to see things in black or white, to divide them into good or bad. The food will then be good or dangerous, a day will be either totally positive or catastrophic. The bulimic crisis is often triggered by all or nothing thinking. The person, convinced that he has now transgressed the iron diet, after eating even small quantities of food, guided by thought, so much so that they have ruined everything, continues in the binge.

Low self-esteem aggravates this aspect of personality. Losing control over the diet in a binge can result in depression, disappointment and anguish. The fact of not being able to maintain a strict diet and indeed having distorted it from bulimic crises makes bulimic patients feel unworthy, guilty and worthless.

In some cases, in Bulimia Nervosa there may be considerable difficulty in controlling and managing impulses. Often they can manifest themselves with behaviors such as making small cuts or burns on the skin, adopting promiscuous sexual behavior, using alcohol or drugs, putting themselves in dangerous situations.

Medical Complications

The physical complications of Bulimia Nervosa are related to compensatory behaviors. Vomiting and improper use of laxatives and diuretics can cause various physical complications. Frequent vomiting can have serious consequences. It can cause an electrolyte imbalance, i.e. a modification of body fluids and electrolytes, such as sodium and potassium.

The most serious complication is hypokalaemia, a reduction in the level of potassium. It can cause hypochloremia and changes in heart rhythm, up to cardiac arrest. The most frequent symptoms of an electrolyte imbalance are dizziness, thirst, water retention, fatigue and apathy. These changes are reversible and disappear when the person stops vomiting. Loss of gastric juice through vomiting can lead to metabolic alkalosis and metabolic acidosis. Vomiting in the long run irreversibly erodes the tooth enamel, especially the inside of the front teeth. In some people who induce vomiting there is an enlargement of the salivary glands. It may happen that the swelling of the glands causes an enlargement of the face, which may suggest that the body has also enlarged, increasing the concern for the weight and body shape.

Reflux esophagitis is a medical condition characterized by the presence of lesions of the esophageal mucosa secondary to retrograde reflux of gastric contents. In people who use their fingers to induce vomiting, small wounds may be present above the knuckles of the hand, initially they are abrasions and then become scars. The mechanical stimulation of vomiting can cause superficial wounds in the back of the throat that can lead to infections. Sore throats and hoarseness are frequent. Vomiting can rarely cause lacerations or bleeding to the esophagus. However, if a certain amount of fresh blood appears in the vomit, a medical examination should be immediately requested to exclude a laceration in the stomach.

Obesity

Obesity is a chronic disease caused by an excess of fat mass distributed differently in the various body areas. To talk about obesity, excess weight must exceed 20% of the ideal weight for height. The simplest and most used parameter to define the degree of obesity is the Body Mass Index and height.

Obesity is not defined univocally. The common orientation is that above a certain body weight it should be considered a chronic pathology like diabetes or high blood pressure. Obese subjects appear to have a reduced life expectancy and a quality of the same compromised.

The adolescent period constitutes a delicate moment for the obese subject. About 75% of cases are a condition that begins before six years of age. However the symptoms occur at any age.

Overweight is perceived as a lack of will, gluttony, little regard for one's health and aesthetics. They use the consumer-food item as an illusory promise to replace the vacuum, but without obtaining anything, just satisfaction. The obese subject accumulates within himself an unlimited amount of food until he feels suffocated.

The body is a prison, it is not felt as one's own, and this armor serves as a shield, as a paradoxical defense against the demands of the other. There is an attempt to anesthetize emotions through an apparent physical enjoyment.

In filling up with everything, one does not experience the emptiness which is what produces thought, desire, and creative acts. The fullness tries to fill the anguish of the void, but it leads to the anguish of a fullness that suffocates and cancels the subject.

Advices for those who suffer from Obesity

Obesity does not pose a direct threat to the life of the individual, except in cases where there is an excess of weight greater than 60%. Certainly, however, it is still compromising the quality of life of the subjects affected. Indirectly it can cause death, since it involves a whole series of serious medical complications.

The currently applicable therapeutic measures must elicit active patient participation in order to be truly effective. Obviously, this participation must be motivated by the recognition of a dissatisfaction linked to the malaise experienced before and after binge eating. It could be boredom, loneliness, the depressive void, which often follows the act of eating, and aesthetic concerns.

This awareness often occurs in adolescence, when the motivation for change is so high that it leads to a greater probability of success. This change does not take place by resorting to a DIY restrictive diet. It is widely recognized that the restriction is a cause of loss of control and therefore of binge eating. This entails a vicious circle of failures that feed low self-esteem, shame, depression, inability to control oneself.

It is necessary to contact a specialist, or better yet a specialized center in which a program that goes beyond the diet is implemented. It is important to look at the person with their experiences, their beliefs, and possibly act on a psychological, educational and behavioral level.

Psychotherapy and Obesity

A serious treatment of obesity should be based both on an assessment of eating behavior and on a cognitive-behavioral program.

Long-term success will be more likely if weight loss will result from a change in lifestyle and dysfunctional behaviors that determine the establishment and maintenance of obesity.

The weight loss diet alone is more likely to recur, with the regaining of the lost pounds, 90-95% of cases. Instead, the goal must be to achieve and maintain a modest but manageable weight loss to improve health conditions.

For this reason, the treatment should also include an educational program aimed at changing eating behavior, promoting motor activity and changing body weight.

The patient should be actively involved in all phases of therapy, informed, educated, supported as in a rehabilitation process. The drastic diet inevitably leads to loss of control with a consequent unscheduled or controlled calorie intake.

Instead, the goal is precisely the acquisition of the ability to control itself, which is achieved by replacing the rigid control with a schedule that also provides for the previously programmed transgression. By managing the diet you are able to experience the pleasantness of control.

Feeling the pleasure of being able to control yourself allows you to get out of failures and guilt. It is a long, difficult path, but possible through the management of a program entrusted to multiple operators who take care of the person as a whole.

Pharmacological therapy and Obesity

To complete the discussion, it seems appropriate to specify that obesity therapy often involves the administration of drugs. Clearly we are talking about particularly serious cases, above all of a mere support to the therapeutic measures exposed so far, which represent the cornerstone of the cure. The drugs used belong to three classes, of the thyroid hormones, diuretics, psychotropics and anorexants. Obviously the use of do-it-yourself is strongly discouraged. The drugs must be administered only under strict medical supervision, also because their uncontrolled intake can lead to very serious damage.

3. BINGE EATING DISORDER

The Binge Eating Disorder, BED, is a disorder characterized by the presence of bulimic crises in the absence of inappropriate compensation behaviors for weight control.

People with Binge Eating Disorder are rarely recognized. They are mistakenly confused with other overweight or obese people, or worse with bulimic ones.

Even those who suffer from uncontrolled eating disorder experience a sense of shame and dissatisfaction with their body, even if an ideal of extreme thinness is not necessarily pursued. They feel a deep sense of discomfort in losing control with food, but unlike obese subjects, they give excessive weight or body figure to assess themselves.

What is the Binge Eating Disorder?

The Binge Eating Disorder, BED is the eating disorder characterized by recurrent episodes of binge eating always accompanied by a feeling of loss of weight control.

Compared to other patients with eating disorders, subjects with uncontrolled feeding disorder have on average a greater weight, a greater frequency of overweight or obesity. Often people with Binge Eating Disorder visit the centers for the treatment of obesity, but compared to patients with obesity they report a greater presence of psychiatric symptoms, in particular depression, anxiety and personality disorders.

Those who suffer from Binge Eating Disorder experienced a sense of shame and dissatisfaction with their body, even if an ideal of extreme thinness is not necessarily pursued. They feel a deep sense of discomfort in losing control with food, but they do not always give excessive weight or body figure to assess themselves. Like people with obesity, people with BED can be discriminated against by others because of their physical condition.

Those with this eating disorder feel dissatisfied, lacking self-esteem, disgusted with themselves and depressed. In certain very serious cases, the pathology of uncontrolled feeding disorder degenerates into cases of self-harm and instinct to suicide.

Debut of the Binge Eating Disorder

Binge Eating Disorder is a disorder that shares some psychopathological aspects with other eating disorders and is almost always associated with obesity. The study of the subject's personality with BED appears useful to etiology science, the sector that deals with researching the causes of the phenomena. In recent decades, numerous researches have stimulated many questions for which further studies are required to provide the appropriate answers. Generally speaking, these are studies on why certain events or processes occur and on the reasons behind certain events.

Binge Eating Disorder typically begins in adolescence or early adulthood, but can also begin in late adulthood. It can appear at any age, affects both genders, with a greater prevalence in male persons. Those affected by it come to the attention of the clinician usually later than individuals with nervous bulimia. Often it is not associated with an emotional discomfort and a diet is usually required as a first intervention, after the numerous and often unsuccessful DIY diets.

In patients with Binge Eating Disorders often, incongruous diets or their failure represent the event that triggers a binge. In this case, however, it is the negative emotions related to the deprivation of the pleasure of food or to the finding of the difficulty in losing weight to induce to exceed in nutrition. Intolerance to negative emotions is definitely an important psychopathological construct for this disorder.

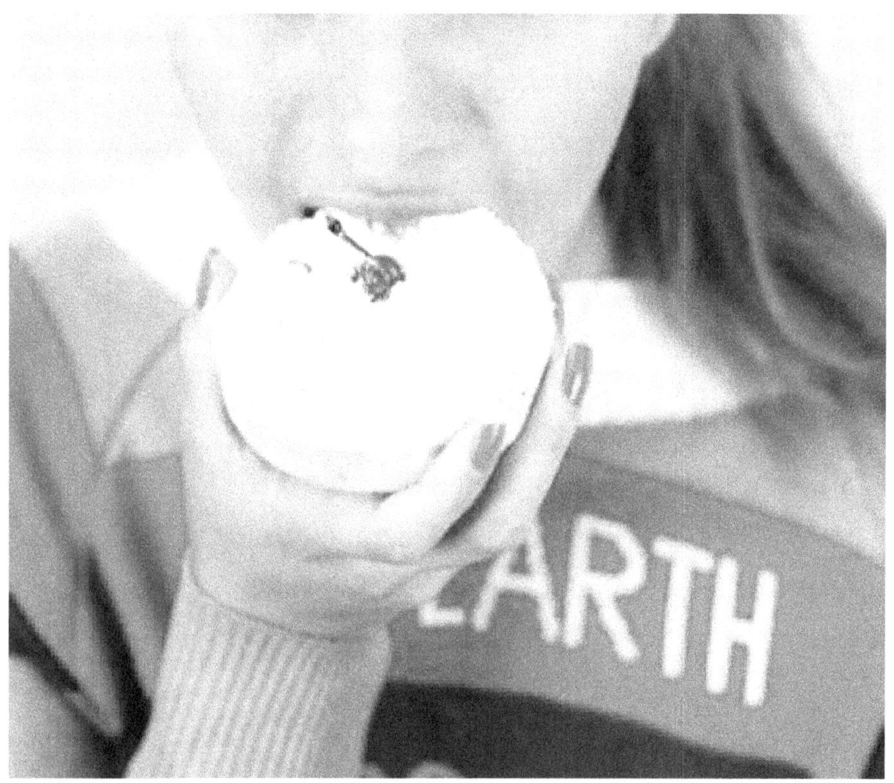

It appears to be recurrent in families, which may reflect genetic influences. There are several studies on risk factors and binge triggers, but none offer completely comprehensive answers. It should be underlined, however, the fact that in addition to genetic factors, neuroendocrine and social factors also appear to be involved. The difficult experiences of childhood life, the presence of depressive disorders in the parents, the tendency to obesity and the repeated exposure to negative comments regarding the form, weight and mode of feeding would seem to play a central role for a reliable diagnosis.

The disorder by BEG occurs in normal weight, overweight and obese individuals. In binge eating, binges are not followed by elimination or compensation practices such as vomiting or purges. Those who have been suffering from it for a long time or in a serious way are unavoidable to experience overweight or obesity. Beyond the psychic discomfort that the person suffering from BED is experiencing, the obesity or overweight condition he may experience will also lead to cardiological, respiratory disorders, typical of obesity.

Developing phases of the Binge Eating Disorder

Individuals with Binge Eating Disorder feed differently than obese or bulimic patients. It is the attitude towards food that is different in these patients. For them, food is an uncomfortable ally, capable of consoling in the saddest moments and gratifying in those of joy, which at the same time leaves behind the guilt of the binge and an unpleasant residue of unnecessary pounds.

A peculiar characteristic of the subject affected is represented by the behavior after the binge. It does not take an active attitude, aimed at restoring the antecedent state, but the passivity, discouragement and sense of inevitability of one's destiny prevails. There is almost never an attempt to remedy the incident that goes beyond good intentions, destined to be regularly disregarded. This attitude is closer to the attitude of a depressed patient than one suffering from eating disorders.

It often emerges that people with uncontrolled eating disorder experience greater levels of anxiety and depression, as well as greater dissatisfaction with their bodies. However, sometimes Binge Eating Disorder patients report binge eating even after positive emotions. The inability to manage emotions leads to excess in uncontrolled nutrition. Binge eating thus becomes the final common response to different emotions, to more disparate moments and events, capable of soothing any discomfort.

An episode of binge eating is defined as eating significantly more food over a certain period of time than most individuals would eat at the same time and in similar circumstances. An episode of excessive consumption of food must be accompanied by the feeling of losing control to be considered a binge episode. These binge episodes are normally characterized by marked discomfort.

Diagnostic criteria of the BED

Those affected by BED implement a series of behaviors that act as clear alarm bells. People suffering from this eating disorder tend to binge or ingest a significant amount of food very quickly. Many patients eat large quantities of food even if they do not feel absolutely hungry and, often and willingly, eat meals alone for the shame of showing up in public.

An episode of uncontrolled feeding is characterized by the presence of two factors:

☐ Eat, in a defined period of time, for example two hours, a quantity of food that is decidedly greater than what most people would eat in the same period of time and in the same circumstances;

☐ Feel a feeling that you can't stop eating and can't control what and how much you eat.

Uncontrolled Feeding Episodes

The most frequent symptoms to be able to establish that it is a diagnosis of a disorder are due to the fact of eating large quantities of food much faster than normal to feel unpleasantly full. Eating alone because of the embarrassment of how much you are eating and feeling disgusted with yourself, depressed and guilty about yourself.

Uncontrolled nutrition is not associated with the systematic use of inappropriate compensatory behaviors, such as the use of laxatives, self-induced vomiting, fasting or physical hyperactivity. A key feature is the loss of control during the episode which however varies between people. Some warn themselves long before they start eating, for others there is a gradual evolution and for still others it comes only after they realize they have eaten too much.

There is a close relationship between BED and obesity. In fact, most people with this disorder are obese or overweight. This does not mean, however, that all obese people are affected by Binge Eating Disorder.

Psychological Characteristics

Compared to other patients with eating disorders, people suffering from BED appear to be less symptomatic. Although, compared with other obese patients who do not have an eating disorder, BEDs report greater psychiatric symptoms, in particular depression, anxiety and personality disorders.

They feel a deep sense of discomfort in losing control over food, but they do not always place excessive importance on weight or body figure to evaluate themselves. Often, people with this disorder are teased and discriminated against by others. It is generally thought that their overweight or obesity is due to excessive gluttony and lack of control.

People suffering from BED are aware that their weight is not only a matter of will, but there are important genetic implications. On the other hand, their almost always irregular diet leads them to feel guilty of their own weight and to live with a deep sense of shame. The more frequent bulimic seizures are, the more people with BED may feel depressed and exhibit other psychiatric symptoms. It therefore seems that the weight, the bulimic crises and the mood tone interact with each other, promoting dysfunctional maintenance of the disorder itself.

BED and the Psychobiological Model of Personality

In order to understand the Binge Eating Disorder well, it is interesting to refer to the psychobiological model of the personality. It could prove to be an additional key to understanding the disorder itself and could help explain such a peculiar disorder.

According to this approach there are temperamental and character dimensions, which could constitute a specific personality model of the BED.

In particular, a high activity of Novelty Seeking NS, exploratory factor of the sphere of impulsiveness and aggression, rewards a rapid loss of anger and avoiding the consequent frustration, in avoiding the damage, would correspond to an anxious-depressive spectrum.

On the contrary, a low activity of Self Directness, SD, corresponds to an indicator of fragility, a difficulty in containing a temperament characterized by impulsiveness and a predisposition to develop a personality disorder.

Impulsiveness and compulsiveness, the pillars of the personality of these patients, are the basis of various dysfunctional behaviors. Such features are present, for example, in the diagnosis of borderline and antisocial personality disorder, attention deficit or hyperactivity disorder, impulse control disorders.

From a clinical point of view, the low activity of Self Directness could prove very useful for drawing up a psychotherapeutic project for its treatment.

Characteristics of the BED

The disease is characterized by an alteration of eating habits and by an excessive concern for weight and body shapes. The medical complications observed in patients with BED are generally related to the presence of obesity, such as cardiovascular, metabolic problems, such as diabetes and dyslipidema, osteo-articular, gastric-intestinal, respiratory, and difficulty healing from wounds.

The evolution of the BED is little known because of its too recent definition and characterization. Some researchers say that the cure rates are similar to those of Bulimia Nervosa that is about 57%, even if these data need further investigation.

An almost always present feature in those suffering from an eating disorder is the alteration of the body image which can become a real disorder. The perception that the person has of his appearance seems to influence his life more than his real image. The body becomes the theater of a profound suffering experienced by the subject. It is the body that must communicate. The image that refers to the mirror is in their eyes that of a person with too wide hips, with too large thighs and with too large a belly. The evaluation of oneself, in subjects suffering from other eating disorders, depends excessively by the weight and shape of your body. The body becomes the bearer of traumatic, difficult and unbearable experiences.

The Role of Impulsiveness

Binge eating occurs, on average, at least once a week and patients experience difficulties in various areas of their lives. First of all, they feel a sort of social unease, extended to most interpersonal relationships. They perceive a distortion in the vision of their body which feeds a sense of insecurity and inadequacy. They register a certain pressure and stress due to the large amount of time spent on a diet and in some cases, they resort to alcohol or drug abuse. They have difficulty managing moods or expressing their emotions, including anger. Their sense of helplessness is linked to the inability to control their eating behavior and the consequent weight gain.

Compared to other patients with eating disorders, subjects suffering from BED have an average weight, a greater frequency of overweight or obesity.

However, compared to patients with obesity, they report a greater presence of psychiatric symptoms, in particular depression, anxiety and personality disorders. Like people with obesity, people with BEG can be discriminated against by others because of their physical condition.

They feel a deep sense of discomfort in losing control with food, but unlike people with bulimia nervosa, they do not always give excessive weight or body figure to assess themselves.

50% of patients with BEG suffer from major depression, panic disorder and some personality disorders. In fact, the binge eating symptom would compensate for a pervasive sensation of persistent discomfort present at the time of the crisis. A high overweight can contribute to the maintenance and accentuation of the compulsive symptom. It gives back to those who suffer from it a sense of failure, guilt and shame that supports uncontrolled food behavior. During the binge episodes the subject is unaware of what he is doing, so there is a loss of control. Afterwards, they are prey to feelings of disgust.

Personality characteristics of the patients are considered as individual vulnerability factors. They allow those who are carriers of it to be more exposed than others to develop this disorder. The consideration of pathological personality traits in BEDs highlights the problem of co-morbidity, or the association of two or more disorders in the same subject. These are the so-called complex cases of particular importance for both research and clinical practice.

At the clinical level, people who are often impulsive and emotionally unrestrained are observed. Eating disorder is an impulsive-compulsive attempt to regulate feelings perceived as intolerable. In particular, some patients report feelings of despair, an inability to tolerate stress and spasmodic research for an immediate feeling of gratification. The uncontrolled intake of food and its elimination thus constitutes and reinforces itself as a failed self-care.

Considering that this disorder has been recognized only recently, the literature on this topic is not very well known. However, some studies concerning personality have focused on the dimension of impulsivity - compulsiveness.

As can be observed in the disorders that are part of the obsessive-compulsive continuum, in the same way in BED, in order to avoid the emotion of anxiety, an impulse is implemented that can guarantee a fallacious feeling of well-being.

Being able to give in to the impulse, in fact, generates a kind of subjective pleasure even if its consequences can be extremely tearing. The person, therefore, perceives that he cannot resist the urge to eat. Before committing the act, the subject feels an increased sense of tension. Only while he commits the act and then eats, does he experience pleasure and gratification.

However, this mechanism triggers a vicious circle whereby, at a later time, negative experiences come to light that arise mostly in the form of senses of guilt and shame.

BED and Impulsivity

In any case, in general, eating disorders and impulsivity would seem to share the same biological basis. Just as eating disorders could be interpreted in a continuum of serotonergic dysfunction.

Serotonin is an amino acid, naturally produced by specialized cells of the intestine and is known as 5-HT. The effect of 5-HT depends on signaling to target cells on brain tissues. It conditions the mood and promotes feelings of well-being. It also impairs appetite, sleep cycles and pain perception.

In impulsive subjects it has been shown that there is an alteration of the metabolism of serotonin and a reduction in the activity of this neurotransmitter. Interestingly, high levels of 5HT would induce anorexic behavior and obsessive-compulsive behavior. While, low levels of 5HT would produce impulsive behaviors, with loss of control over eating behavior. Consequence that subjects affected by BED would lead to bulimic behavior.

According to the cognitive approach, the patient would be subject to repeated extremes in the judgment of himself and the environment. All black or all white, there is no middle ground. The lack of sufficient self-awareness facilitates the onset and maintenance of extreme behaviors. This produces the alternation of restrictions and binges, such as to re-propose to the individual their inability to lead a balanced existence. The result could be dangerous, since the sense of failure is strengthened even in the face of a small food relapse. In this way, the onset of guilt, the insinuation and the subsequent perpetuation of depressive symptoms is favored.

In particular, impulsivity plays an important role especially in maintaining dysfunctional behavior. Faced with a potential threat, the individual with a strong trait of impulsiveness does not seem to have the cognitive resources necessary to adequately assess the event and identify the most appropriate response. On the contrary, there is a high probability that aggressive behavior will take place to protect or avoid pain. It is a matter of implementing a sudden response in reaction to a stimulus coming from the external environment through a behavioral scramble. The subject uses food behavior as a protection strategy. The method used not only in BED but also in other eating disorders seems to be linked by a single common thread. Illusively, one tries to control and manage one's emotional experience in an attempt that seems to want to reactivate the body with food. In addition to the concomitant presence of addiction to alcohol and drugs, in some subjects with BED there are other behaviors related to impulsiveness such as sexual promiscuity, kleptomania, self-injurious behavior or suicide attempts.

In light of the foregoing, it is pointed out that some features and modalities could compromise the already difficult treatment of these patients. In particular, perfectionism and impulsiveness can affect the treatment of these ailments by hindering the therapeutic alliance.

Acceptance of One's Emotions

Dysfunctional emotional management is one of the main characteristics of eating disorders. The study of the emotional state of patients is a branch that needs to be deepened in order to deal with those who are affected by Binge Eating Disorder with the right competence.

From our analysis it is clear that, in order to effectively deal with the problem of the Binge Eating Disorder, it is necessary to intervene with a psychological path. This path must be aimed at increasing the ability to regulate the emotions of the subjects, starting primarily from the work on accepting their negative emotions.

If the individual denies the possibility of experiencing certain types of emotions, the fact of increasing the emotional awareness in themselves is absolutely insufficient for the solution of their problems. As long as they do not legitimize themselves in their feelings, in fact, their emotional recognition will be worth nothing.

Acceptance of emotions is the fundamental element in order to be able to activate functional regulation strategies, which are not based on compromise but, rather, on addressing and regulating the emotion in place managing the situation that generated it.

In this regard, it may be useful to propose, in a psychological intervention aimed at managing the Binge Eating Disorder that allows you to reach a greater awareness of the emotions you feel, through an attitude of listening to yourself. Accepting emotions through a non-judgmental attitude allows you to accept the experience as it is and evaluate it without stereotyped labels or commonplaces.

Through the possibility of learning to recognize one's own bodily signals, the ability to accept one's emotions is developed without judging them at any cost. This attitude would avoid having to resort to defensive escapes and self-injurious behavior. In this way, we move from an automatic reactivity to the implementation of a response that is more suited to the needs of subjects who show a dysfunctional relationship with food.

Anger and Negative Emotions

Another interesting aspect would be to investigate which emotions are more difficult to accept by subjects who exhibit Binge Eating Disorder behaviors. One of the emotions to highlight is definitely anger. The greatest difficulty in relating is anger, which characterizes subjects with a dysfunctional relationship with food. Anger is experienced as a negative emotion.

Anger is experienced as wrong and not socially acceptable. It cannot have a positive meaning. However, the difference between experiencing anger and engaging in angry behavior is not considered. In this way, one cannot perceive the evolutionary meaning of anger or even experience the specific emotion of anger. It is possible that this particular difficulty in relating to anger is due to external judgment, towards those who are experiencing this relational situation; experiencing anger would, in fact, more easily lead to behaviors that can be misjudged by others.

Being badly judged for an abnormal behavior means having to question one's amiability and validity as individuals. With a view to a future development of a research study, it would be interesting to evaluate the modification of the ability to regulate the emotions of the subjects affected by Binge Eating Disorder following a mainly psychological path. Everything must be based on the enhancement of emotional regulation skills to allow subjects to accept their emotions, whatever they are.

4.PREVENTION AND CAUSE OF THE BINGE EATING DISORDER

Prevention

Prevention includes all those health and non-health interventions that seek to reduce the onset, chronicity and negative consequences of those affected by Binge Eating Disorder.

Prevention interventions are usually divided according to the moment in which they act. Before the onset of the disease and at the first signs of symptoms. It allows an early identification of the subjects concerned, and this one is the most opportune moment to reduce or eliminate the risk factors.

When the disorder is full-blown, the prevention coincides with the treatment of the disorder itself, to prevent patients' possible physical and mental complications.

Primary Prevention

Many scholars have wondered if preventing eating disorders is possible. There are many questions about the possibility of prevention and the answers are not univocal. Numerous studies in the field of eating disorders and their possible causes have led to understanding that there is no single cause for these disorders. Many factors combine to predispose, precipitate and then perpetuate the disorder. These factors are of various types, genetic factors, socio-cultural factors, psychological factors, biological factors.

By definition, primary prevention is possible only when the etiological factors are known and modifiable. If it is possible to intervene on socio-cultural pressures, it is not possible to intervene on genetic factors. It is very important to understand whether primary prevention interventions reduce the incidence of eating disorders. Explaining to someone or a group of people what eating disorders are is even counterproductive and harmful.

Mechanisms of imitation and identification can trigger, as often these serious diseases are idealized. The same automatism is triggered by the testimony of people who have suffered from these problems. For this reason, it is good to be wary of preventive programs based only on information regarding these ailments.

On the contrary, many studies have instead found that interventions that stimulate discussion and the development of a greater critical sense towards the messages of the mass media can be useful. This type of intervention should not deal exclusively with eating disorders, but range more widely on the different problems of one's own experience, the relationships one has with one's body and interpersonal problems.

Other forms of potentially useful intervention could be interventions aimed at people at high risk, or interventions that aim to enhance protective factors, improve self-esteem, problem solving and communication skills.

It is therefore essential to evaluate the effectiveness of the preventive programs before implementing them. In times of rationalization of resources, it is important to invest in interventions of sure efficacy and without potential risks.

Secondary Prevention

Then there is another type of prevention, called secondary, which intervenes on cases as soon as possible with respect to the onset of the disorder. It has been ascertained, at a clinical level, that a treatment undertaken in the early stages of the disease is more effective. However, in the early stages of the disease, the person with an eating disorder does not always understand and admit that he needs help. Also at this level it is therefore important to raise awareness of the environment, starting from the same people interested in the family. The right prevention requires the ability to recognize eating disorders to facilitate the request for help in specialist centers, in general practitioners and specialists for these pathologies.

Food as a Relief from Negative Emotions

Compulsive nutrition is characterized by ingesting large quantities of pleasant foods, in order to alleviate a negative emotional state. This element can also be found, for example, in the symptoms of obsessive-compulsive disorder, from the decrease in the reward from anxiety and stress.

The diminished reward feature is characterized by the loss of motivation for ordinary rewards. The negative feeling derives from the involvement of the stress-related brain systems that are involved in this mechanism, causing irritability and anxiety.

Therefore, when a behavior becomes compulsive, a shift in the factors that motivated it is assumed. Initially the behavior is positively reinforced, later the compulsion could arise from the negative reinforcement mechanisms. Experiences of anxiety and irritability when the reward, that is, the food sought is not available, condition eating disorders that lead to compulsive eating behavior.

As regards nutrition, abstinence from certain foods is configured with a diet. It implies a reduction in the calories ingested, going from highly prohibited foods to an increase in healthier and less palatable foods. Numerous studies have in fact highlighted how the majority of obese subjects, at the beginning of the diet, experience intense sensations of irritability and anxiety. The transition from a food balance rich in calories to a less caloric one leads to a worsening of mood and depressive symptoms. Diet as a stress management strategy highlights that attempting emotional self-healing through comfort food is counterproductive.

The self-induced diet worsens a negative emotional state. Having access to palatable foods after a period of deprivation leads to excessive consumption. This alleviates the discomfort caused by depression and anxiety, but can lead to compulsive nutrition, instead of getting relief from anxiety or stress.

Negative Consequences of Compulsive Nutrition

The last element of compulsive nutrition seems to be the loss of control, due to a deficit in the mechanisms responsible for suppressing inappropriate actions. These deficits likely confer vulnerability to addictive behavior. Stakeholders are encouraged to delay dysfunctional behavior rather than end it.

This lack of inhibitory food control often persists despite the physical, psychological and social complications that lead to uncontrolled nutrition. These subjects often suffer from negative emotions following binges, due to experiences of shame, denial and guilt.

When these negative emotional and physical consequences outweigh the desirable effects of a pleasant food, people often attempt to start a diet, although they often fall back into improper and unhealthy eating habits.

Self-referential Company

It is a new society today, a 2.0 society, of self-care and self-diagnosis. A society in which stereotypes and prejudices are the masters, especially as to regards external beauty. Today, in fact, a body is defined as beautiful only when it is able to wear tight sizes and trendy clothes.

All this has consequences, to look beautiful, you have to be online and follow diets, most often found on websites or by famous people who promote their healthy diet.

Strange diets, accompanied by supplements and pseudo-drugs that guarantee excellent results in a short time. Diets that come from all over the world and that, through a few steps, can be found and available to everyone. The prescription of specialists who calibrate the diet on the person after an accurate medical examination is avoided.

Contentment and satisfaction for one's body have always been topics treated and considered as an obsession. In the beginning, this was mainly visible in the female sex, but today it seems that the male world has adopted this attitude too, but in a different way. The lack of fulfillment for males focuses on a lack or lack of muscles or poorly defined physicality. In women it focuses on thinness or elimination of fat mass. In fact, for these and other reasons, eating disorders such as Bulimia, Anorexia, Vomiting and Binge Eating Disorder mainly affect the female population, even if there are significant exceptions.

Eating disorders are described as pathologies characterized by alterations in eating habits and by excessive concern about one's image, in particular weight and body shapes.

Socio - Cultural Aspects

Social and cultural factors play a very important role in the genesis of food problems and pathologies. The great influence of the media and the continuous representations of models of physical perfection contribute significantly to the increase in cases of eating disorders with a significant and sometimes even devastating impact on adolescents and vulnerable subjects.

Therefore, guided by a distorted perception of their body and not by objective reality, these people obsessively seek perfection, which they identify in the unattainable reference models proposed by the mass media. The compulsive behavioral modalities typical of eating disorders are used to overcome negative states such as anxiety, inadequacy, low self-esteem and desire to please others.

The introduction of social media, has increased our exposure to images of retouched and artificial photos and consequent benchmarks far from reality. Although a direct link with the development of eating disorders is still to be demonstrated, it has been found that the emphasis placed by social media on the image is related to the development of greater anxiety towards the image itself, negatively affecting one's self-esteem.

Studies have shown that women and men who do not deal with the models conveyed by the mass media have a more positive perception of their image, as well as a better acceptance of their body shape.

In the face of globalized models of reference, the contradictory presence of mass media messages linked to food over-stimulation is associated. The result is a dissonant social communication which can in some predisposed subjects contribute to the onset and development of dysfunctional eating behaviors, with serious repercussions on health.

It is possible to do prevention of eating disorders in numerous ways. With the correct and appropriate knowledge on the topic of eating disorders, it is possible to convey more appropriate messages through a real social communication.

In this way, risk factors and the probability of spreading the disease can be transformed into preventive factors, making a significant contribution to tackling a problem of social relevance and promoting the adoption of healthy attitudes with respect to the perception of one's own body weight and shape.

Prevention Factors

With a view to the prevention of problems and disorders of eating behavior in adolescents, a fundamental role is played by educational action. The info about the nutritional properties of foods should be always considered, indicate the healthy foods to be taken and those that should be avoided. Since young age, at school, the competences for developing an individual capacity for critical evaluation should be transmitted. The educational purpose is to make consumers aware and immunized from the negative effects that many commercial messages can convey. In this way, we would become aware consumers rather than passive subjects who mechanically are exposed on business adverts on a daily basis.

At the basis of these disorders there are a series of factors that lead the person to delude himself that he can shift the control over food that one thinks he does not have over his life. Very often, one feels excessively worried about the judgment of others, influenced most of the time by the inability to establish meaningful social and personal relationships.

Factors Responsible for the Binge Eating Disorder

A sort of pendulum has often oscillated in the search for the factors responsible for eating disorders, going from organic to psychological and environmental factors. Today, the scientific community tends to propose multifactorial models for eating behavior disorders. It agrees that there is no single cause but a concomitance of factors that can differently interact with each other in favoring their appearance and perpetuation.

To have a correct idea about the development dynamics of the BED, a long series of factors that refer to a bio-psycho-social perspective must be kept in mind. This means that in the onset of an eating behavior disorder, factors that create a sort of predisposition or vulnerability come to interact. Genetic factors interact with cultural factors, on which other triggering factors act and precipitate the situation, which otherwise could remain latent. This in turn creates the conditions for the disease to perpetuate itself.

Predisposing Factors

Of the predisposing factors we will examine only some specific characteristics. Individual characteristics are some individual notes shared by people suffering from BED. These elements contribute to preparing a ground on which the disturbance of eating behavior can be grafted.

Registry Component

The first element is of a registry type. Teenagers are most vulnerable and most affected. Adolescence is an extremely delicate period of transition between childhood addiction and the autonomy of the adult phase. The eating disorder can arise from the inability to cope with these changes, the fear of maturity and all the requests and responsibilities it entails. In a certain sense, illness is a means, a way of staying or returning to children, in a protected situation both on the physical and on the emotional, cognitive and social levels.

Among the psychological factors, the idealization of thinness seems relevant. Skinny is good, fat is bad. This is the strong message that society sends. Girls know that men look at their bodies and are educated to be looked at. Having a body that respects the prevailing aesthetic canons becomes a sort of necessity for social relations.

Perfectionism

Generally there are personality traits characterized by perfectionism. These are ambitious people, with excellent results at school and in the activities they undertake, which show a commitment and tenacity often considered proof of great maturity and responsibility. This attitude of dedication and sacrifice almost always hides low self-esteem and profound personal insecurity, which expresses the fear of not being accepted by others for what you are.

The person thinks that he will be accepted only on condition that he gives his best without the slightest stretch mark. In people who get sick these traits are pushed to exasperation, any commitment that has nothing to do with the study or the activity on which it is invested is eliminated. The fear of disappointment and failure is great. The judgment of others is assessed as the only way to estimate one's worth. Many people are absolutely convinced that they are not as others would like them and they adapt to this idea by trying in every way to meet the expectations of others. They go on an obsessive search to trace the presence of a pathological perfectionism, due to an evaluation of themselves dependent by the achievement of certain very demanding and self-imposed personal standards. The judgment of others is considered the only way to estimate one's value.

Linked to perfectionism is a particular type of thought, called dichotomous thinking. Jumping from one extreme to another, there are no middle grounds, indeed half measures are not even considered. It is, therefore, a dichotomous personality, which moves between all or nothing, between moral contradictions, of thought and behavior. The obsessive lives on logic, in rationality and order, concepts that mix poorly with emotions.

In their relationship with others, they tend to lead, to make arrangements to be able to control better, and when they say something they actually give orders for being meticulously executed; only in this way do they satisfy their need for tranquility. They has no faith in anyone, delegating would be a risk, if they did, control and rules would fail.

Even emotions are subject to strict control, because if shown they are synonymous with weakness and vulnerability. They experience anger whenever they are unable to maintain control of their physical and interpersonal environment, however, they hardly express it directly, because they concentrate on what the others want, how to control addiction.

Before the disease becomes evident in many of these people traits of obsession, anxiety and depression are found. It is possible that these aspects are consequent to the state of malnutrition. The obsessive aspects, however, often seem to be pre-existing to the onset of the eating disorder.

Role of the family

The role of the family in the onset of an eating disorder has often been emphasized also inappropriately. The various theories that have dealt with this aspect have often referred to a disturbed relationship between mother and daughter. A particular configuration of family dynamics presents an overprotective, intrusive dominant mother and an absent father. In reality it is impossible to know whether a particular family climate is the cause rather than a consequence of the disturbance. It would be strange to imagine that in front of a daughter suffering from eating disorders, a parent does not become overprotective and that this does not cause a great increase in family tension.

What appears from the expanded observations of families with a BED-affected component is that there are a variety of different family situations and it is difficult to find common denominators. Today the idea that there is a typical family that favors the onset of anorexia is no longer accepted.

A separate consideration must be spent for those families in which there is a particular attention to the issues of physical appearance and nutrition. It is likely that a family atmosphere in which these aspects are emphasized could lead to the construction of a polarized self image on the external aspect. However, even in this case, there is no evidence that eating disorders occur more frequently in contexts of this type. Significant studies have shown that a high body dissatisfaction in parents favors a similar attitude.

The predisposing factors include, for example, pregnancy complications and perinatal damage, the presence of family members who suffer or have suffered from an eating disorder, have low self-esteem, interpersonal difficulties, body dissatisfaction and the use of low calorie diets. Risk factors are those factors that are capable of increasing the vulnerability to develop a particular disorder.

At the basis of these disorders there are a series of factors that lead the person to delude themselves that they can shift the control over food that one thinks they do not have over their life. Very often, one feels excessively worried about the judgment of others, influenced most of the time by the inability to establish meaningful social and personal relationships. Disorders of this kind can also occur following situations of severe stress or trauma.

Triggering Factors

The triggering factors are events that can determine the onset of the disorder in people who have a predisposition. They can be stressful or traumatic events such as bereavement, abuse, illness, family conflict, breaking an important relationship, changing school or city. In some cases it is not always easy to identify triggering events.

The fate of a person who presents a vulnerability to an eating disorder can be different depending on whether or not he or she encounters so-called triggering factors in his or her life which favor and determine the appearance of the actual disorder.

It is believed that undertaking a weight loss diet even in conditions of modest overweight, if there is a predisposition to the disorder, represents a crucial trigger. This obviously does not mean that all people who start a diet will experience an eating disorder. The combination of triggers seems to be the formula necessary for the manifestation of the disorder.

Sometimes the onset of weight gain is not associated with situations of body dissatisfaction but with adolescent problems, such as the impetuous changes that are observed during puberty development. The detachment from the family and the beginning or the end of an emotional relationship could be considered as other triggers. These are always events that tend to increase the difficulties encountered in terms of relationship skills and of one's autonomy and self-esteem, the change of residence, the loss of friends, the occurrence of physical or psychological harassment. At other times these are situations related to difficult and negative moments in life such as the death of a relative, a friend, an illness, a family crisis.

Usual Voluntary Actions

The current models for the search for triggers focus attention on three elements in particular. As for the first aspect, it must be remembered that the formation of a habit is the final result of an adaptive learning process.

Voluntary actions become habitual through reinforcement mechanisms. Overeating is the result of a learned habit. Environmental stimulus related to food, known as conditioned reinforcements, can sturdy increase the desire to eat even in the absence of food itself or in the absence of physiological needs related to hunger.

Through repeated pairing of a stimulus, a conditioned and unconditional stimulus with food, the learned stimulus becomes a salient incentive. It thus causes intense impulses to obtain the associated reward. It also acts as a conditioned reinforcement that contributes to maintaining the desire to seek food.

Habits can be considered compulsive when they persist despite devaluation. In compulsive nutrition, the inability to adapt eating behavior based on the motivational value of the result, may reflect a compulsive habit.

Compulsive behavior is hypothesized to reflect a maladaptive habit that previously constituted flexible and voluntary behavior.

Habits are formed through repeated action until the stimulus-response association interrupts the purpose of the behavior. For example, the search for a particular food represents a motivation to perform the action.

In some research it has been highlighted how compulsive behavior can be generated by a conflict or a stressful situation. In this case, this behavior tends to be characterized by its compulsive nature even when the triggering stimuli are absent. In other words, once this behavior has taken root, a sort of euphoric satisfaction is produced which produces addiction, comparable in all respects to substance dependence.

Maintenance Factors

The food restriction and the consequent decrease in weight, are all factors that over time promote depression, irritability and dissatisfaction with your body.

These factors, through a closed circuit mechanism, can induce a further food restriction, aimed at improving one's self-esteem.

It is very important to take these aspects into due consideration since, especially in the most serious and long-lasting situations, interventions should be aimed precisely at reducing these factors. In the impossibility of finding a precise cause to be removed, the most effective intervention is represented by the modification of those elements that keep the disorder alive.

Thought Aspects

Thought aspects are important initially. The ideas on weight and body shapes push the person to formulate a single thought regarding the physical aspect. This is followed by all those actions that can lead to the achievement of this goal. The intervention, in this case, must aim to question these defined dysfunctional assumptions. Often these ideas are reinforced from the outside, as it is not uncommon to find someone who compliments a normal weight who goes on a diet.

Over time, however, external reinforcement tends to decrease and the most important maintenance factor becomes the symptomatology determined by fasting. People who undergo a reduced diet, after a first phase characterized by euphoria and hyperactivity, develop a complex series of symptoms and signs that involve organic, behavioral and psychic aspects.

There are often important changes on the emotional level and depressive and irritability states emerge. Sometimes even more serious psychiatric manifestations can be found. A tendency to social isolation is often evident, amplified by the objective difficulties that the person suffering from BED in dating other people.

Friends, after a first moment, in which they encouraged the diet, become perplexed in the face of excessive weight gain and do not share their concerns about food. Furthermore, being together often involves convivial moments such as eating pizza or ice-cream. On these occasions, those suffering from BED only experience anxiety, embarrassment, desire for self-exclusion.

The onset of psychiatric symptomatology, anxiety, depression, irritability and the tendency to close in on themselves place the person in a condition in which any relationship is difficult, and even the acceptance of external help is problematic.

The person with an eating disorder has learned that controlling food is a powerful tool for controlling his anxieties and fear. Any attempt to reduce control can trigger a crisis of anxiety and depression.

After the initial phase, there is a decrease in the ability to concentrate, which often has to do with the need to increase any type of commitment. There is also a regression of the form of thought which becomes similar to that of the child, linked to the concrete data of everyday life and unable to elaborate hypotheses on the future. A situation occurs in which apathy, poor ability to concentrate are accompanied in a framework that tends to perpetuate the basic disorder.

As far as people with BED are concerned, the main factor of maintenance is the dominant thought of the binge which often becomes a diversion, a filler and an outlet that can appear more manageable against a crisis of anxiety and depression.

Over time, the person suffering from BED develops an inability to distinguish the different biological stimuli of hunger and satiety and to perceive to correctly manage anxiety, anger, loneliness and sadness.

They delude themselves that their bulimic eating behavior is a way to quell moments of anxiety and tension. Awareness of the resulting benefits is often minimal. The person who wants a cure is convinced that they want to change, but as the change looks forward they can realize that their determination is not so strong. The consequences are represented by feelings of guilt and personal disregard that can frustrate the drive to overcome the problem.

In these situations, a review of the motivation for treatment appears useful. In this sense it has always been said that bulimic behavior is experienced as negative and unpleasant.

The person suffering from BED would like to avoid binges but to assume a restrictive and controlled eating behavior, aimed at achieving that much desired body weight, but almost always too excessive, so he cannot maintain it.

The consequence would be above all in the fact that in the case of bulimia there is a more frequent request for help. Often the greatest willingness to care found in bulimia is only apparent. Beyond the declarations and also the real awareness of the person, the binge as abhorred is the means to quell anxiety. The moment when you give in to the temptation of food becomes a way to let go, to release tension, to give yourself forbidden food, to remove any negative thoughts. The binge is carefully planned, ensuring an adequate supply of food and eliminating any disturbing element.

Family Dynamics

Another factor of maintenance can be represented by family dynamics. The beginning of the problem can induce behaviors that, although perfectly understandable, unfortunately tend to perpetuate the disturbance.

The emergence of an overprotective attitude has the effect of reducing the autonomy of the subject. A situation of regression of the entire family is therefore created at a stage in which the parents had to deal completely with the feeding of the child.

If we consider that the engine of eating disorders is often represented by the fear of growing and becoming self-employed, it becomes evident how this situation can be more coherent with the maintenance of the disease. One modality that has proved particularly interesting for parents is that of self-help groups, where parents exchange experiences by providing mutual support. However a more careful reading of the situation can allow us to understand that these advantageous situations are nothing more than protective and defensive modalities that are assumed to face fear and difficulties.

5. CURE AND THERAPY

Proper Diagnostic Evaluation

For the treatment of eating disorders, it is important to contact specialist centers ideally expert with these problems. This will permit differential diagnosis to be made. The only way to understand if you suffer from a real eating disorder is to carry out all the necessary specialist psychological, psychiatric, internal and nutritional assessments. This is the only way to receive the correct information on the treatment to be followed.

Not all problems concerning eating behavior are real eating disorders.

A differential diagnosis allows us to understand if we are faced with other psychiatric diseases, such as depression or phobias, or with internal diseases such as celiac disease or endocrine problems.

The initial evaluation also has many other important objectives. First of all, it is the moment when a relationship of trust is established between the patient and the doctor. In the evaluation phase, all the information needed by the therapist is collected in order to understand which is the most appropriate path to follow.

The diagnostic evaluation generally lasts 2-4 visits made by a psychologist or psychiatrist and investigates the eating habits and attitudes regarding the patient's food and body. The social and family situation, school or work functioning and interpersonal relationships are assessed. In addition to the interview, the survey can also be conducted with interviews and questionnaires.

If the danger of medical complications is glimpsed, the diagnostic evaluation must be completed by an internal-nutritional examination. Finally, if the patient is under age, a visit for the parents is also indicated to complete the diagnostic picture. The point of view of the family members serves to establish an atmosphere of collaboration, as the family represents a point of trust even if the patient were to refuse or abandon therapy.

Care of the Binge Eating Disorder

An effective treatment of the Binge Eating Disorder disorder must take into consideration the medical-internal part, the nutritional part and the more strictly psychological part.

The main problem is therefore the close connection between emotion and food. Food becomes a tool to anesthetize negative emotions. At the same time, however, the Binge conducts lead to feelings of guilt and unease. This creates a vicious circle harmful to the patient's physical and mental health.

This is a psychological and emotional disorder that encloses a very painful personal situation.

For most people with BED, the awareness of having a problem is low and the fear of facing a change is very strong. Eating without control, extreme diets, can be seen by the person suffering from BED not so much as a disturbance, but rather as a solution to their problems. This disturbance is so pervasive that it leads to the illusion of being able to keep other life problems away. In fact, many problems are caused by the eating disorder itself.

This is the reason why many people with eating disorders, especially in the early stages of the disease, do not ask for help or even refuse a therapeutic approach. Many epidemiological studies have found that people with BED ask for therapeutic help. In any case, the therapeutic contact allows in these cases to open a dialogue and to monitor any complications, both medical and psychological.

If a person with an eating disorder is not yet able to undertake a real treatment, a motivational path is usually started. That is, a psychological path that aims to bring the person to desire change and healing.

Being motivated to change means feeling an unease that gives the awareness of getting involved and the courage to ask for help. A collaboration between different professional figures who deal in an integrated way with these disorders that can be psychiatric with important psychopathological manifestations.

The most effective approach for the treatment of eating disorders is the multidisciplinary and integrated one.

How to Choose the Treatment

When a person with eating disorders arrives in a specialized facility, a correct and careful diagnostic evaluation with a multidisciplinary and integrated approach for more or less intensive treatment is essential.

It is always a good rule to start, except for specific contraindications, from the less intensive treatment, i.e. outpatient treatment, because it interferes less with the social life of the person. Only in cases where outpatient treatment has not worked will more intensive treatment be used, such as semi-residential day-hospital treatment.

The choice to carry out a therapeutic program in hospitalization regime is made when there are medical complications, such as a very high frequency of bulimic crises, improper use of drugs, multi-impulsivity, self-aggressive behavior, high suicidal risk and failure to previous treatments.

The most suitable treatment for the person must be chosen together with a trusted therapist after a thorough diagnostic evaluation. The factors to be considered are the type of disorder, the physical situation, the presence of complications, the duration of the disease, the age, the person's expectations, previous therapeutic experiences and the characteristics of the patient's personalities.

Nutritional Treatment

The performance of the nutritional program will ensure that you are able to prevent loss of control over your diet or sudden weight gains. This point is very important and must be shared with patients who obviously have many fears and concerns in facing food and changing habits.

The aim of nutritional rehabilitation is to gradually restore correct nutrition by inserting the foods considered taboo in a guided and gradual way and contrasting the trend towards dietary restriction. Therefore, both the quantity of food and the quality problems are tackled, including those considered fattening and therefore phobic. The path must be carefully guided taking into account the patient's fears and duration of illness. Discomfort may initially arise due to digestive difficulties resulting from a prolonged restriction.

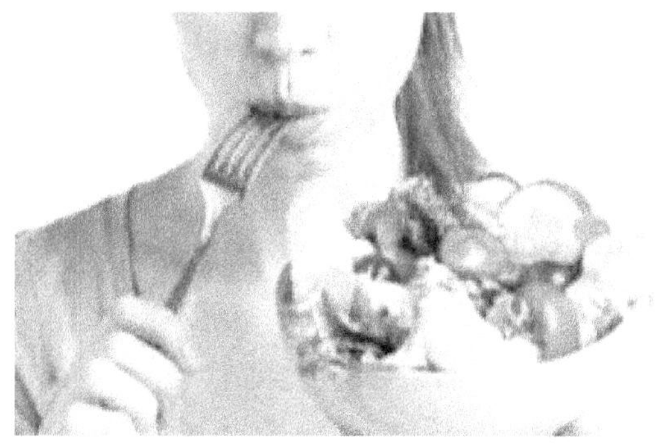

The food program is divided into 3 main meals plus 1 or 2 snacks. In outpatient treatment, the division of meals throughout the day, the portions of the courses and the type of food to be included are agreed with the therapist, tested at home, verified and discussed in the next meeting.

The Pharmacological Treatment

Pharmacological treatments are based on antidepressants, serotonergic, that is, serotonin reuptake inhibitors such as citalopram or paroxetine. They work correctly, but they have the defect that after a few months the results go down. Having reached this last stage, the subject is able to limit binge eating. Obviously, if in the meantime the personality or the experience evolves positively, all the causes at the origin of the depression will also be removed, making the compensation mechanism underlying the Binge Eating Disorder useless.

The use of drugs is linked to the observation that other psychopathologies are often associated with these disorders, such as depressive and obsessive-compulsive disorders. For this reason, the most frequently used drugs are antidepressant drugs with mainly serotonergic action. The pharmacological treatment of eating disorders should never be considered as the main treatment, but always as a supportive treatment for psychotherapeutic or psychoeducational work.

In bulimia nervosa, antidepressant therapy has shown specific efficacy in reducing bulimic symptoms and in reducing associated psychic symptoms, such as depression, obsessive symptoms and impulsivity. The long-term efficacy of antidepressant therapy remains poorly understood and the clinical impression is that even in bulimia nervosa antidepressant treatment can only be effective in association with psychotherapeutic treatments. The use of mood stabilizing drugs, associated with antidepressant therapy, can be useful in the treatment of anorexia nervosa and bulimia nervosa when they are associated with multi-impulsive characteristics.

Psychological Treatment

Psychological treatments are based on the control of food intake, on the variation of eating habits, up to a real food consciousness.

The psychological treatment proposed for eating disorders considers the presence of incorrect or distorted knowledge about food and one's body as the main responsible for pathological attitudes and eating behaviors. Behaviors such as food restriction, avoidance and weight and body control behaviors are in turn factors for maintaining distorted cognitions. In psychological therapy, therefore, both incorrect eating behaviors and related cognitive style are addressed.

The Cognitive-Behavioral Model

TCB model essentially consists of three main phases. In the first phase, the patient is given information on the disorder, the aim is to reduce binge eating and regularize the frequency and composition of meals with alternative activities to bulimic crises.

In the second phase, the goal is to improve the quality and quantity of nutrition, to face the idea of a diet, to recognize risky situations and to practice problem solving exercises.

In the third phase, the results obtained are consolidated and the topic of relapse prevention is addressed. A very useful technique is the use of the food diary, in which the mode and quantity of nutrition, the emotions and beliefs related to food are recorded by the patient. Through this self-monitoring, patients learn to recognize and avoid risky situations and behaviors, obviously after having analyzed everything with the therapist.

In reality, the TCB uses a global approach called transdiagnostic. In a first phase of the treatment, it focuses on managing the acute phase of the eating disorder and subsequently the therapy plans to address all the problems associated with the eating disorder, family difficulties, relationships and the development of a fragile self-esteem.

Cognitive Behavioral Therapy can be individual or group. The group approach has been successfully used for bulimia nervosa and in uncontrolled feeding disorder. Review and meta-analysis studies have highlighted the effectiveness of these treatments on the evolution of symptoms and on the improvement of the psychopathological picture. The sense of shame, of secrecy that characterizes bulimic crises, interpersonal difficulties, isolation and low self-esteem lead the subject to increase feelings of guilt and a sense of inadequacy. The group can become a place of reflection, comparison and transformation.

Interpersonal Psychotherapy

Developed by Klerman in 1994 for the treatment of depression, it has been extended to the treatment of bulimia nervosa and BED. This addresses the difficulties of interpersonal relationships designed at the basis of eating disorders.

Interpersonal psychotherapy involves a first phase in which the focus of the treatment is identified. A thematic area is addressed by choosing from 4 categories, difficulties in forging and maintaining significant ties, conflicts with relatives and friends, difficulties in role changes and unprocessed bereavements.

In the next phase the patient takes on a more active role and is invited to talk about his current difficulties and to experiment with new relationship models to relate them to the focus of the problem that has been previously identified to prepare the patient for the problems they will face in the future.

Psychoanalytic Psychotherapy

Psychoanalysis assumes that the symptoms are the expression of unconscious conflicts. Psychoanalytic psychotherapy acts mainly on what are considered to be the predisposing factors for dietary pathology. Its goal is to allow the maintenance of the results achieved through the analysis and resolution of internal conflicts and interpersonal problems. Through introspection, the patient discovers and analyzes these conflicts.

The psychoanalytic approach is useful if the physical and psychic consequences of the symptoms are not such as to prevent psychological work. It is therefore advisable to undertake this type of therapy only once the weight has been recovered or the frequency of bulimic crises has improved in order to address the underlying psychological problems.

Food Psychoeducation

Psychoeducation is an educational technique that aims to raise awareness of the mechanisms by which a particular disorder has arisen, is maintained and can be cured. It takes into account patients' rights to be fully informed and improves adherence to treatments because it involves the patient in the therapeutic choices.

As for eating disorders, very often wrong and distorted information and beliefs circulate about the caloric content of food. Psychoeducational techniques consist in providing correct information on the properties of nutrients, on the metabolic functioning, on the biological effects of restrictive diets, on the reasons of amenorrhea, on the relationship between weight loss and physical and psychological symptoms.

In some initial and non-serious cases, psychoeducation, together with some nutritional advice, can in itself lead to a remission of the symptoms. The absence of at least one regular meal a day or the use of compensatory methods shows the need for more specific help. Isolation and poor social support are other factors that make the success of a purely psychoeducational intervention difficult. In general, therefore, psychoeducation can be considered a very useful therapeutic technique, but which must be associated with other therapeutic interventions.

Family Therapy

Family therapy is an important part of treatment, as it involves and works with families. The goal of family therapy is to promote change, with sessions supervised by a family therapist.

Family therapy must be considered when a malfunction is observed within a family. It helps to highlight problems concerning the general ability of the family to respond to emotions under stress. This form of therapy can be useful to eliminate those potentially lethal situations for the BED, of which the family very often contributes to the cause despite being unaware of it.

An advanced version of this therapy is called the Maudsley Method. This family-based treatment focuses on involving parents as an active role in the recovery process of the child from eating disorders. This would include parental guidance in helping their child eat balanced and healthy meals and prevent deviant behavior.

Several studies suggest the usefulness of treatments aimed at family members with the aim of improving knowledge related to the disease and its treatment and to decrease the family burden and excessive emotional involvement.

Family therapies can help parents better understand the pathological aspects of their child's behavior and can be helpful in interrupting the vicious circle of the disease.

The goal of family therapies is not to search for the causes of the disease but to have possible co-therapists within the family, to better contribute to the success of the treatment. Often these are apparently simple tasks, such as easing the tension at mealtimes, but which require good control so that it is better to behave in one way rather than another. This is the psychoeducational approach that involves providing information on eating disorders and their treatments in order to improve collaboration in treatment.

Cognitive Rehabilitation Therapy

Cognitive rehabilitation therapy is a treatment that is born for people resistant to treatments. It is an intervention that can be used both as a pre-treatment program and as an additional module to cognitive-behavioral psychotherapies.

It is an intervention that consists of mental exercises aimed at improving cognitive strategies. The assumptions on which the program is based are constituted by the idea that the brain and the process of information are not given once and for all, but that they are able to change throughout life if subjected to specific training.

The purpose of the treatment is to help the patient acquire a series of strategies that facilitate the acquisition of greater thinking flexibility. The patient will be put in a position to adopt a more global style of thinking, against the tendency towards excessive attention to detail.

It is a slightly different approach from the classic psychotherapeutic interventions. It mainly addresses how the patient thinks and not the content of thought. No emphasis is placed on the food symptoms manifested by the person, but attention is paid to the thought processes through the use of simple and specific cognitive exercises different and far from nutrition and weight. This generally reduces the patient's resistance by improving adherence to therapy (compliance). It consists of mental exercises aimed at improving cognitive strategies, thinking skills and the acquisition of information through practice, to promote a reflection on thinking styles. It helps explore new thinking strategies in everyday life.

Self-help Group

By reading and using self-help manuals on the market on eating disorders, the patient tries to solve their problem on their own.

A number of people suffering from eating disorders gather in groups according to the rules of anonymous alcoholics to fight the eating disorder, usually the BED more rarely than the bulimia nervosa.

Reading and using self-help manuals are combined with the support of a professional. The patient can also be guided in this form of therapy by the general practitioner, a dietician or a social worker. There are studies that have proven the effectiveness of pure and guided self-help in patients with non-serious forms of eating disorder and there are several manuals.

CONCLUSION

This book is mainly aimed at subjects affected by Binge Eating Disorder, to stimulate them to adopt more balanced lifestyles aimed at psychophysical well-being. At the same time, we wanted to give indications to many people on how to avoid health risks deriving from incorrect information on eating disorders.

Eating disorders are psychiatric conditions that use the body as a means of expressing frustrations. For this reason, it is extremely important to implement a diagnostic approach that takes into consideration the organic, psychological and social endocrine components.

Patients who are affected by these disorders often have very serious organic complications. Generally, it is the symptoms that lead the patient, driven by family members, to a first contact with the doctor. In most cases these subjects diminish the entire symptomatological spectrum.

The treatment of patients with these pathologies varies based on the type of disorder and the level of impairment of the patient's health. The integration of multiple specialists in the therapeutic planning and management of these patients remains the most suitable form of intervention. With these patients, the first thing to do is to establish a very close exchange of trust before starting a therapeutic relationship.

The therapist will conduct an accurate and detailed history of the subject's history to understand the individual factors related to the development of the disorder. The clinical experiences reported by the therapists come to the conclusion that the patients' experiences, their traumas are considered risk factors predisposing to the development of psychiatric and food disorders. Therapy will be characterized by a remarkable flexibility of a program, which gradually adapts to the intellectual abilities and experiences passed by the various patients.

In fact, the main objective of this work concerns the origin and evolutionary path of BED. The most effective contrast to this disorder is given by the possibility of resorting to a global therapeutic program, which focuses on both memories and situations present, which cause emotional distress.

In patients with eating disorders, there is a strong tendency to isolate and avoid contact with others. The traumatic experience can upset the existence of an individual causing negative feelings of distrust towards themselves and towards others and altering emotional patterns.

Appropriate therapies help the patient to construct information constructively and to experience what he feels within himself. Guilt and shame are progressively transformed into adequate responsibility of an adult being, who make their choices confidently. The solution of the disorder is achieved through the stimulation of the patient's innate self-healing processes. The information processing mechanism is physiologically designed to solve psychological disorders in the same way that the rest of the body is equipped to heal a physical injury.

When the patient has worked out his frustrations, he will also be able to recall the positive events that have occurred, which allow him to redefine himself as a person of positive abilities, with a past and a future. The patient's evaluation of himself changes, thanks to the internal emotion processing system that is stimulated, so that the healthy nucleus that is already present can emerge.

Cognitive behavioral therapy is today the most effective treatment for the treatment of these disorders. It regulates the eating style through psycho educational encounters, which make it possible to know useful information to deal with and resolve the disorder and the prevention of possible relapses.

Patients with eating disorders become aware of their abilities and leave the sense of emptiness to increase their self-control. Interpersonal psychotherapy allows the reworking of past and present events that cause disturbance, teach patients to value the past, to plan the future and manage stress without resorting to binge eating.

Through these programs, people suffering from Binge Eating Disorder can learn to manage their emotions and thoughts and can develop a healthy relationship with food.